Imaging Strategy
A Guide for Clinicians

Imaging Strategy
A Guide for Clinicians

BOB BURY
Consultant Radiologist
Leeds General Infirmary;
Senior Clinical Lecturer in Radiology
University of Leeds

and

RICHARD FOWLER
Consultant Radiologist
Leeds General Infirmary;
Senior Clinical Lecturer in Radiology
University of Leeds

OXFORD NEW YORK TOKYO
OXFORD UNIVERSITY PRESS
1992

Oxford University Press, Walton Street, Oxford OX2 6DP

Oxford New York Toronto
Delhi Bombay Calcutta Madras Karachi
Kuala Lumpur Singapore Hong Kong Tokyo
Nairobi Dar es Salaam Cape Town
Melbourne Auckland Madrid
and associated companies in
Berlin Ibadan

Oxford is a trade mark of Oxford University Press

Published in the United States
by Oxford University Press, Inc. New York

© *R. Bury and R.C. Fowler, 1992*

A catalogue record for this book is available from the British Library

Library of Congress Cataloging in Publication Data
Bury, R. F. (Robert F.)
Imaging strategy : a guide for clinicians / Bob Bury and Richard Fowler.
(Oxford medical publications)
Includes bibliographical references and index.
1. Diagnostic imaging—Handbooks, manuals, etc.   2. Radiography, Medical—
Handbooks, manuals, etc.   I. Fowler, Richard, Dr.   II. Title.   III. Series
[DNLM: 1. Diagnostic Imaging—handbooks.   WN 39 B975i]
RC78.7.D53B87   1992   616.07'57—dc20   92-22706
ISBN 0-19-262063-0 (pbk.)
ISBN 0-19-262323-0 (hbk.)

Typeset by Downdell, Oxford
Printed in Great Britain
by Dotesios Ltd
Trowbridge, Wiltshire

Preface

Even in the most enlightened centres of learning there is still very little radiological teaching in the undergraduate medical syllabus. As a result, most junior doctors (and, dare we say it, quite a few senior ones) know little of what goes on in radiology departments, and are confused by the array of imaging techniques now on offer. Our book attempts to remedy this ignorance. The aim is not to teach image interpretation, but to give advice on how to make the most efficient use of the imaging department, avoid unnecessary investigations, and ensure that a diagnosis is reached as soon as possible. The first four chapters advise on the use of the department, put into perspective the hazards of imaging (notably that due to radiation), give brief details of the imaging techniques available, and explain what some of the commonly requested investigations involve from the patient's point of view. This section, particularly the first chapter, contains the general principles which are necessary if you are to make good use of the more specific factual information given in the second part of the book, which deals with the different body systems in turn.

Wherever possible, the systematic chapters deal first with those clinical presentations which rank as emergencies. Here the junior member of the firm may well be on his or her own at least initially, and will need to make an appropriate choice of imaging investigation. Just as important, they will need to recognize those situations where imaging has no part to play. We then consider the 'cold' investigation of patients on the ward or in the outpatient clinic. This pragmatic approach has resulted in an apparently arbitrary and idiosyncratic selection of topics, but we felt that it was important to concentrate on the common conditions likely to confront the junior hospital doctor, using the patient's presenting symptoms and signs as a framework wherever possible. In some chapters this format is inappropriate, and we have modified the layout.

You will find the phrase 'consult your radiologist' cropping up at frequent intervals. The aim is to encourage you to make the best use of available radiological expertise—a few minutes spent discussing a difficult patient can help to avoid unnecessary investigations and facilitates prompt diagnosis and treatment. Another piece of advice which recurs throughout the book is 'follow your local protocol'. Although this may look like prevarication on our part, it is simply a recognition of the fact that there are areas where a number of acceptable imaging strategies exist, and all we can offer are general guidelines.

We hope that the book will be of use to medical students and junior hospital staff and even to some of the more senior hospital doctors. Although there is a limit to how many 'pocket guides' the overworked houseperson can be expected to carry around, with any luck there will be a copy on the shelf in the ward office or casualty department when it is needed.

Leeds
1992
B. B.
R. F.

Acknowledgements

We would like to thank our radiological colleagues for their helpful comments and advice, in particular, Rosemary Arthur, Graham Bonsor, Alan Chalmers, Paul Chennells, Delia Martinez, Geoff Parkin, and Keith Simpkins. Thanks are also due to Gillian Rishworth for typing the manuscript, and to the Medical Photography Department at Leeds General Infirmary for the illustrations.

Finally, we wish to thank Lin and Sarah, our wives, who tell us that without their cheerful support and forbearance this book could not have been completed.

Contents

1

Using the radiology department

Requesting an examination

The request for an imaging procedure initiates a consultation between radiologist and clinician which may have a crucial bearing on the well-being of the patient. There are three elements in the referral process which you should consider.

1. *Is imaging necessary?*

It has been estimated (NRPB/RCR 1990) that approximately 20 per cent of radiological investigations are unnecessary—this is probably a conservative estimate. As you write the request, ask yourself two questions: 'what will I do if the suspected abnormality is present?' and 'what will I do if the result is negative?' If the answer is the same in each case, then think twice (at least) about the need for imaging.

However, when talking about the influence of an investigation on management, we need to interpret the word 'management' in its widest sense. The value of a normal result is now generally acknowledged, and it may even be acceptable to perform an investigation just to reassure a patient. Remember though, the acceptability of 'for reassurance' on the request form will depend on the cost, radiation dose or invasiveness of the examination in question. While a chest X-ray might be appropriate, a radiculogram would not.

2. *Which examination?*

Twenty years ago there was only a limited choice, but advances in radiology have resulted in many more imaging methods becoming available, and some of the older procedures are now obsolete. This has been good for patients, but has made life more difficult for clinicians faced with an ever increasing array of imaging techniques. Our chief aim in writing this book is to make the choice easier, and reduce the number of inappropriate requests. A few general principles are worth outlining at this stage:

(a) Define a question which you want the investigation to answer, and write it on the request form. Resist the urge to fire off a salvo of requests in the hope that one of them will hit the target. In particular, decide what sort of information you are after—it will seldom be necessary to know everything about the organ or system under investigation, and this can influence the choice of examination.

For example, if a patient has long-standing obstructive uropathy affecting one kidney, and nephrectomy is contemplated, you will choose a renogram to give you the *functional* information that you need (i.e. is the kidney still obstructed, how much is it contributing to overall function) rather than an IVU which will give you mainly *anatomical* information. If on the other hand your patient has been shown to have a renal carcinoma, you may want a CT scan to give you the *anatomical* information you need to stage the tumour prior to surgery.

Conversely, there will be little point in requesting two different investigations which give the same type of information. For example, both CT and ultrasound give a cross-sectional anatomical image, and it is wasteful to request them both in the initial investigation of a patient.

(b) Choose the examination most likely to give you the answer. Although it is laudable to choose the cheapest, least invasive and

most readily available investigation first, there is no point performing an array of plain film procedures if you know you are going to need a CT scan eventually.

(c) If, after considering a and b, you still have a choice, go for the test which involves the lowest radiation dose to the patient. With the advent of ultrasound and MRI, it will sometimes be possible to avoid the use of ionising radiation altogether.

(d) Consider the patient. Most doctors have no idea what is involved in, for instance, a barium enema and this is one of the reasons for writing this book. Many of the investigations we perform involve discomfort and some carry a significant morbidity. Even an IVU, often requested with hardly a second thought, can be a very uncomfortable procedure, even for those patients who do not have a true contrast reaction (p. 15). You need to keep this in mind when deciding if imaging is justified for a particular patient. Remember that an examination which would pose no problem for a fit thirty-year-old might be a major physical and mental trial for a frail elderly patient, and the diagnostic reward considerably reduced.

(e) Make use of previous films. Without these it may be impossible for the radiologist to give an accurate interpretation of the current findings, and previous studies often show that further investigation is unnecessary. Of course, films are sometimes lost irretrievably, but it is never acceptable to repeat an examination just because they are not immediately to hand. A recent report (NRPB/RCR 1990) found that in orthopaedic clinics 30 per cent of radiographs were only performed because previous films had not been made available.

(f) When in doubt, consult the radiologist! Patients do not always present with straightforward problems, and there will often be doubt as to the best imaging strategy. We are always happy to talk to clinicians, and it is much better for all concerned (especially the patient) if discussions take place before

a string of unhelpful examinations have been performed, rather than afterwards.

• *Royal College of Radiologists' Guidelines:* The RCR have produced a small booklet entitled *Making the best use of a department of radiology* (RCR 1989). This gives guidelines to the sensible use of twelve common radiological investigations which between them account for 95 per cent of the work in most departments. Many radiologists are distributing it to their clinicians, but if yours is too mean, it is well worth a pound (1990 price) of your own money. Apart from anything else, it will reduce the need to request examinations for medico-legal reasons—if you can show that your decision not to send a patient to X-ray was in accordance with the advice of the Royal College, you should be on safe ground.

3. *The request form*

Radiologists frequently complain, often with good cause, about the quality of the requests they receive. The request form may be the only communication between the referring clinician and the person performing or reporting the investigation, and so it needs to be properly completed. Several points deserve attention.

(a) Sign the request. Most investigations involve radiation or other hazards for the patient, and each request should be signed by the requesting clinician. Stacks of pre-signed cards should not be left in wards and outpatient clinics for nurses to fill in—one day someone will make a really silly request and it will be your name at the bottom. Even worse, this practice leads to the un-necessary irradiation of patients, which carries considerable medico-legal implications at a time when the public are becoming much more aware of radiation hazards.

Your signature, like most, is almost certainly illegible. In a large hospital the radiologist cannot be expected to recognize the paw marks of the ever-changing house staff, so print your name alongside the signature, and give your bleep number. Then if we need further clarification of some point in the patient's history before proceeding we can contact you easily, saving time and worry for the patient.

(b) Make sure the patient details are adequate and correct. Every year radiologists perform investigations on the wrong patients because of errors in completing this part of the form. Quite apart from the medico-legal aspects, there are good clinical reasons for requiring this information. The age and sex of the patient can often affect the differential diagnosis of a particular radiological finding, for example in a patient with a bone tumour. We also need to know where the patient was referred from—the most exquisite and erudite report is no use if we do not know where to send it.

(c) Give sufficient clinical information. The lack of clinical detail is the radiologist's most frequent cause for complaint with request forms. Many radiological signs are non-specific—they can be the result of more than one pathological process, and it may not be possible to come up with a useful report unless the request gives the clinical context. Failure to do this can result in the incorrect interpretation of the examination findings, and may lead to unnecessary additional examinations.

(d) Write legibly—it does not matter how conscientiously the request is completed if the radiologist cannot read it.

(e) Urgent requests. Contact the radiologist directly if you feel a patient requires urgent investigation—this enables us to fit the patient in as soon as possible, and we will be able to advise on the most appropriate imaging sequence.

(f) Out-of-hours requests. Radiology is no longer a nine-to-five speciality, and we do our stint on-call like anyone else. If you have a patient who you think would benefit from a special procedure out of hours then we are always ready to discuss the case and carry out any examination we agree is necessary.

However, most of the on-call work done in radiology departments consists of plain film procedures performed by the duty
radiographer. Much of this is necessary, but a great deal of it
could easily wait until the following morning. For example, a
patient admitted in the middle of the night with an exacerbation
of his chronic obstructive airways disease will seldom need an
immediate chest X-ray.

Unnecessary imaging procedures performed out of hours are
more expensive than the same examination performed during
the working day, and as the work is carried out unsupervised the
appropriate views are not always obtained.

'Portable, please' Large numbers of requests are received for
mobile radiography on the wards, mostly chest X-rays, and
again these are not always indicated. Mobile examination is only
justified if the patient is genuinely unable to come to the department, the investigation cannot wait until they are fit enough to
do so, and the result is likely to influence management. The
apparatus used is inferior in several respects to the departmental
machinery, and it is often impossible to achieve optimum
positioning of the patient. Ward radiography of any part of the
body other than the chest is seldom helpful. In particular, it is
difficult to obtain a satisfactory plain abdominal film on the
ward except in the slimmest of patients. Lest we sound wholly
negative on the subject of ward investigations, it is worth pointing out that a mobile ultrasound examination of a sick patient
can be very useful indeed, and will often be the procedure of
choice.

Preparing the patient

If you are to get the best out of your imaging department, then
patients need to be properly prepared for their examinations.
There are two aspects to this preparation, physical and mental.

1. *Physical preparation*

For many of the procedures we carry out, the patient will need to undergo some sort of physical preparation. There are a number of reasons for this, but usually it is either to give us the best chance of obtaining a diagnostic result, or for the patient's comfort and safety. An example of the former is the fairly rigorous purgation required for a double contrast barium enema, and of the latter the advice to fast a patient for a short period prior to any examination involving the intravenous injection of contrast medium, in order to minimize the risk of vomiting/aspiration. Details of the preparation needed for individual procedures will be given at the appropriate points in the text. Failure to prepare patients may result in a non-diagnostic examination which needs to be repeated, and in the worst case may damage their health.

2. *Mental preparation*

This is something which doctors are very bad at—we tend to underestimate the anxiety experienced by patients referred for even the simplest form of diagnostic imaging. There may be a considerable delay between your decision that imaging is required and the actual appointment, particularly for outpatients. During this period, the patient will conjure up all sorts of visions of what is involved, and friends and relations will be only too happy to supply lurid and inaccurate details concerning their own experiences (or more likely those of a third party relayed by several intermediaries).

Much of this anxiety can be avoided by a few words of explanation at the time you make the decision to refer, and here we have a problem. Most clinicians, junior or senior, have very little idea of what is involved for the patient in any but the simplest of plain film examinations. For example, clinicians send in referrals for barium studies with little understanding of the mechanics of the investigation or the preparation required, and are therefore in no position to answer any questions their patients might have.

Although radiologists are largely to blame for this state of affairs, there are things that you can do yourself to remedy matters. The first step is to read (and, we hope, buy) this book, but you should also pester your local radiologist to let you see a few examinations in progress, preferably on your own patients. It is likely that once you have seen a difficult barium enema performed on a frail distressed eighty-year-old, your referral rate will fall. An even more effective way to ensure this would be to insist that all junior medical staff undergo an enema themselves, including the preparation, but that might be a little excessive.

Using the results of imaging

1. *The X-ray report*

The report on an imaging procedure should be concise, intelligible, and should answer the question you asked. If the radiologist is unable to answer your question, there should be some indication of any further imaging investigation which might help. We do not always achieve this ideal, but we do try. If you are not clear about the meaning of the report, do not be afraid to ask; as pointed out above, the request is not always a gem of lucidity, and we may have misunderstood the clinical problem. Most of us go to great pains to avoid sitting on the fence, and try to give a definitive answer wherever possible, accepting that we will sometimes be wrong. When we are wrong, it is important that you tell us, as this is the only way that we can improve our service.

If a report is needed urgently, indicate at the time the request is made that you need a quick report. This avoids the problem of a harrassed secretary struggling to find it in the middle of a dictaphone tape when the radiologist has gone off to another hospital, or to the golf course. Try to avoid ringing up for the result before the patient has arrived for the examination, it makes us cross.

2. *Choosing a test and utilising the result*

There is no such thing as a perfect investigation, in imaging or in any other branch of diagnosis, and even a 'good' test will be unhelpful if it is used for inappropriate clinical indications, or in the wrong patient population. A number of parameters are used in describing the accuracy and usefulness of diagnostic tests, and these are defined in Table 1.1, while Table 1.2 shows how the predictive value of a test varies with the prevalence of the disease in the population.

When deciding whether an investigation is likely to be useful in a particular patient, 'prevalence' is not a very useful concept, but what you should have is some idea of the prior probability

Table 1.1   Definition of terms used in assessing the utility of clinical tests

$$\text{SENSITIVITY} = \frac{\text{True positives}}{\text{True positives} + \text{false negatives}}$$

$$\text{SPECIFICITY} = \frac{\text{True negatives}}{\text{True negatives} + \text{false positives}}$$

POSITIVE PREDICTIVE VALUE (likelihood that a patient with a positive test actually has the disease)

$$= \frac{\text{True positives}}{\text{True positives} + \text{false positives}}$$

NEGATIVE PREDICTIVE VALUE (likelihood that a patient who tests negative is actually disease-free)

$$= \frac{\text{True negatives}}{\text{True negatives} + \text{false negatives}}$$

Table 1.2 Examples showing the effect of prevalence or prior probability of disease on the predictive value of an investigation

---

sensitivity of test = **90%**
specificity of test = **90%**

1. Prevalence (or prior probability of disease) 10%:
In population of **1000**:
    100 have the disease, and **90** (90%) are test +ve.
    900 are disease free, of whom **90** (10%) are test +ve.
    ∴ of **180** positive results, **90** are TP, and **90** are FP
    i.e. **positive predictive value** is only **50%**
but:
    of **100** with disease, **10** (10%) are test −ve
    of **900** without disease, **810** (90%) are test −ve
    ∴ of **820** −ve results, **810** are TN, and **10** are FN
    i.e. **negative predictive value** is **99%**

2. Prevalence 50%:
    positive predictive value = 90%
    negative predictive value = 90%

3. If prevalence is 80% the values would be **97%** and **70%** respectively.

---

that the patient has the disease, which amounts to the same thing. As well as this prior probability, you should consider how much harm would be done by failing to diagnose the disease, how effective the likely treatment is, and whether the treatment itself carries significant risk. For example, if you are looking for a test to diagnose a condition which invariably requires hazardous surgery, you will wish to avoid false positive results which lead to an unnecessary operation, and will be prepared to risk a few false negatives (i.e. you will be prepared to sacrifice sensitivity for specificity).

Two further clinical examples may help. Suppose you have a patient with chest pain, and analysis of such factors as age, sex, symptom pattern, and ECG findings add up to an 80 per cent pre-test probability that he has ischaemic heart disease. There would be little point subjecting such a patient to an expensive and potentially hazardous thallium scan (p. 142). If it was positive it would only increase an already high probability by a few per cent, and in a patient with a pre-test probability of disease as high as this, a negative result would have a relatively low predictive value, and would probably not make you reconsider your diagnosis. The scan will have much more value in patients where there is serious doubt about the diagnosis for some reason, and where more evidence is required before progressing to invasive examinations such as coronary angiography and major surgical treatment.

At the other end of the spectrum, if you wish to pick up small breast cancers in asymptomatic women, it is no good choosing manual palpation as your test method. Its lack of sensitivity would result in many false negatives, and in a screening test you want to be reasonably certain that a negative result means absence of disease, (i.e. you want a high negative predictive value). So you choose the infinitely more sensitive method of mammography, accepting a higher incidence of false positives, which will hopefully be revealed as such in the further testing carried out following recall. Then of course, you start to worry about the psychological morbidity resulting from the recall of women who turn out not to have malignant disease, not to mention the financial and opportunity costs of the screening programme; but then, no-one said it was easy.

Finally, remember that even when the positive predictive value of a test is 100 per cent, if the result will not influence treatment, or if there is no effective treatment available, then you will almost certainly be wasting everyone's time and money by requesting the investigation, and the patient will not thank you for it.

2

Hazards of imaging

Causes of morbidity in the radiology department include the radiation itself, the drugs used during the course of some investigations, and the invasive component of interventional procedures. Of these, the radiation hazard is the most important from the point of view of the clinician.

The radiation hazard

Patients are becoming more aware of the hazards of modern medicine in general, and of radiation in particular. The risks of ionizing radiation affect both the patient and their children if the gonads or a developing fetus are included in the radiation field.

The largest man-made contribution to population dose comes from the medical use of radiation (Table 2.1), and yet most of the adverse publicity centres on the nuclear power and reprocessing industry. It has been estimated that a 1.5 per cent reduction in medical exposure would have the same effect on population dose as closing down the whole nuclear power industry, and this level of reduction could easily be achieved without detriment to patient care—hence the importance of radiation protection.

The nature of the hazard

The patient subjected to irradiation is at risk of developing malignant disease in the irradiated area; the latent period before tumours arise can be 20 years or more. The fetus affected by

Table 2.1 Sources of human exposure to ionizing radiation

Natural

Radon	55%
Cosmic radiation	8%
Terrestrial (rocks and soil)	8%
Internal (e.g. ^{40}K in body tissues)	11%

Man-made

Medical uses	15%
Consumer products	3%
Other (includes occupational, nuclear industry, fallout etc.)	<1%

---

irradiation *in utero* may be born with congenital abnormalities, particularly mental defects, and may also be at risk of developing childhood malignancy. Egg and sperm cells are even more sensitive to the harmful effects of radiation than the developing fetus.

The magnitude of the hazard

No one knows how dangerous small doses of radiation are. All the figures that are quoted are derived by extrapolation from the damage done by high dose irradiation, either given therapeutically, or acquired in the nuclear explosions at Hiroshima and Nagasaki. The risk estimates assume that there is no threshold dose for the harmful effects of radiation: that is, there is no safe dose. They also assume a more or less linear relationship between dose and the likelihood of damage occurring.

Keeping the risk in perspective. Whatever the level of risk might be, we do know that it is so small compared to the 'natural' incidence of malignancy and birth defects that it is unlikely that anyone will ever be able to prove that a particular patient has suffered damage from the sort of dose received in the course of a diagnostic investigation. If the worst happens and an early pregnancy is inadvertently irradiated, it will seldom be an indication for termination. If in doubt, consult your radiologist.

The effect of age. Young tissues are more sensitive to the effects of radiation, and young patients have their whole lives ahead of them in which to manifest any of its delayed effects, such as malignancy. This is why we give so much attention to keeping doses down when investigating children—the advent of ultrasound has been particularly helpful in reducing the use of ionizing radiation in paediatric imaging. Older patients are less sensitive to radiation, and are unlikely to live long enough to manifest the adverse effects of radiation received during their latter years.

Reducing the risk

Safety first. Because of all this uncertainty, we err on the side of safety by assuming the worst case. For radiation workers and members of the public there are dose limits laid down for annual exposure. There are no dose limits set for patients—we use the lowest dose possible consistent with reaching a diagnosis, balancing the potential adverse effects against the dangers inherent in leaving disease undiagnosed and untreated. This is the ALARA (as low as reasonably achievable) principle. You, as a clinician, can help keep patient doses down by ensuring that imaging procedures are only requested when there is clinical justification, and that any old films in your possession are made available to the radiologist (see Chapter 1).

The '28 day rule'. For reasons mentioned above, we take particular care to avoid irradiating a developing fetus. Until recently we had the 'ten day rule' which attempted to limit non-urgent investigations involving irradiation of the pelvis of women of childbearing age to the ten days following a period. The assumption was that for patients with a regular cycle, there was little or no possibility of an early fetus being present before ovulation had occurred.

In practice the 'rule' (it was really only a recommendation) was widely misapplied, and resulted in the unnecessary postponement of many investigations for minimal real benefit. It is now known that there is little chance of damage to a fetus before the 14th or 15th day of gestation (i.e. 28 days after the last period), and so most patients will have missed a period and know they may be pregnant before their child is at risk.

Female patients of childbearing age are now simply asked if there is any chance of their being pregnant. Only if the answer is 'yes' will thought be given to postponing the examination until after the next period—even then, this will only be considered if the investigation is non-urgent, and the uterus will be included in the irradiated field. Radiography of the chest or extremities, properly performed, should not result in significant exposure of the uterus or ovaries.

Remember that egg and sperm cells are probably more sensitive than the fetus to radiation damage, and so the only sensible rule is to avoid irradiating them wherever possible.

Contrast media reactions

Iodinated water-soluble contrast media have now been in use for many years, and given the number of injections administered, often to sick patients, there is no doubt that they are much safer than many other drugs used in clinical practice. Nevertheless, there are risks. True reactions range from mild urticarial rashes to circulatory collapse and death.

Even for the majority of patients who suffer no reaction, the administration of contrast media can be less than enjoyable. Frequent side effects of intravenous use include an unpleasant feeling of warmth, metallic taste, nausea, and sometimes vomiting. Some adverse reactions are due to the high osmolality of the media, and others to an incompletely understood anaphylactoid reaction. Most reactions are unpredictable.

                    Imaging strategy

The magnitude of the risk

The mortality rate for the intravenous use of contrast media in different series varies between 1 in 15 000 and 1 in 117 000 (Grainger and Dawson, 1990) but is usually quoted at around 1 in 40 000. This may not sound a lot, but the fact that there is any mortality at all is worth bearing in mind when requesting investigations requiring the use of contrast media. Even mild or moderate reactions, although not posing any threat to life, can be extremely uncomfortable for patients, requiring the administration of parenteral antihistamines or steroids.

Reducing the risk

High risk groups. Although it has already been said that reactions are somewhat unpredictable, there is evidence that they are more commonly encountered in patients with an atopic history and it makes sense to avoid contrast injection if possible in these patients, or to use the newer low osmolality media (see below). There is evidence that a course of steroid treatment can reduce the incidence of reactions in atopic patients, but it needs to be started at least 12 hours in advance of the investigation. Contrast injection should be avoided in patients who have suffered a previous severe reaction: in these cases, discuss the imaging strategy with your radiologist.

New contrast media. Many of the adverse effects of conventional contrast media are related to their high osmolality (up to eight times that of plasma). Over the past ten years or so, a range of low osmolar media have been developed, and although these have not been proven to reduce mortality, we do know that they lower the risk of reactions by a factor of approximately five (more for severe reactions). They also result in a much lower incidence of the minor side-effects mentioned above.

So why not use the new media for all patients? Well, inevitably they cost more than the conventional pharmaceuticals—up to 15 times as much depending on the manufacturer and country.

Switching to the use of low osmolar media in the USA would cost an estimated one billion dollars per year—approximately three million dollars per life saved at 1988 prices (Jacobson and Rosenquist, 1988). At the moment, UK radiologists tend to use the new media for most arteriographic procedures, and for intravenous injections in high risk patients (see Table 2.2). It is likely that conventional media will eventually be completely replaced by low osmolality formulations, the speed of the change being governed by cost-benefit considerations.

Table 2.2 High risk groups in which low osmolar contrast media are indicated (Grainger, 1984)

---

1. Increased risk of anaphylactoid reactions (e.g. rashes, bronchospasm, cardio-respiratory collapse etc.) in patients with:

> history of allergy
> asthma
> previous significant contrast medium reaction

2. Increased risk from the hyperosmolar effects of conventional contrast media in the following conditions and groups of patients:

> infants and small children
> cardiac impairment
> renal failure
> diabetes
> myeloma
> sickle-cell disease

Patients in group 2 must not be dehydrated prior to contrast injection (this is no longer considered necessary in any case, see p. 33)

Other drugs

We use other drugs in radiological procedures, for example, Buscopan and glucagon in barium work; frusemide, ACE inhibitors, and dipyridamole in nuclear medicine. The responsibility for ensuring that these are used safely lies with the radiologist. Any adjustments that might need to be made to the patient's pre-existing medication should be notified to you as part of the preparation for the examination.

Hazards of interventional procedures

Radiologists are now becoming more involved in the treatment of patients, and we regularly undertake procedures such as abscess drainage, biopsies, angioplasty, and embolization which would previously have required open surgery (see Chapter 16). These procedures are not without their hazards, but they are usually considerably safer, and less traumatic, than the surgical alternative. Again, you may be involved in the preparation of these patients; for example by ensuring that coagulation parameters are normal, and by controlling hypertension.

3

Review of
imaging techniques

We grew up in the days, not so long ago, when 'X-ray department' meant just that—there wasn't anything else. Times change, and now we work in the 'Department of Clinical Radiology' with its 'modalities' and 'workstations' as well as the good old-fashioned lightbox and magnifying glass. The advent of new techniques such as nuclear medicine, ultrasound, computed tomography and now magnetic resonance imaging have expanded the scope of radiology enormously, and radiologists now take a much more active role in patient management. At the same time, it has become much more difficult for clinicians to keep up to date with current trends in imaging, and many are unfamiliar with the nature of the new techniques.

As a clinician you need to know something about the new technology in order to rationalize your requests and to answer any questions your patients might have (they will have read all about it in the Readers' Digest!). The aim of this chapter is to give a quick guide to imaging methods, so that when a subsequent chapter recommends a particular technique, you will know what is involved. The amount of space given to each topic does not reflect its usefulness—most of the work in our departments consists of plain radiography, but we skate over this fairly lightly, as most clinicians will already know as much as they need to know about such elementary matters.

Imaging using ionizing radiation

Plain films

Plain film radiography is still the bread and butter work of most departments, and many patients will never require the more sophisticated techniques covered later.

The film, sandwiched between two sheets of card impregnated with a substance which fluoresces when it absorbs X-rays, is enclosed in a rigid cassette. The relevant part of the patient is placed between the X-ray tube and the cassette, and the exposure made. Films, screens and cassettes are available in a range of shapes and sizes to match the region under examination.

Tomography

Not to be confused with computed tomography (see below). Because a radiograph is a two dimensional representation of a three dimensional object, the region of interest can be obscured by tissues lying in front of or behind it. Simple tomography circumvents this problem by allowing the X-ray tube and cassette to move in opposite directions in a fixed relationship to each other during the course of the exposure. This is achieved by linking them with a rigid bar. As a result, only the structures lying in the plane of the pivot remain sharply defined, everything above or below this level is blurred out. The level of the pivot, and hence the imaging plane, can be adjusted. This technique is often used in IVUs when the renal outline is obscured by faeces in the colon, and also in patients with suspected lesions on the CXR.

Fluoroscopy/fluorography (screening)

All your patients coming along for barium meals and enemas will be subjected to fluoroscopy, as will any other patient in whom we need to follow the progress of contrast material through the body, in angiography for example.

The principle is exactly the same as plain film radiography, but instead of using photographic film, the transmitted radiation falls on to a fluorescent screen, and the faintly visible image is amplified by an image intensifier and displayed on a monitor in real time for daylight viewing (fluoroscopy). Representative frames can be captured on film (fluorography) or the whole examination can be recorded on cine film or videotape.

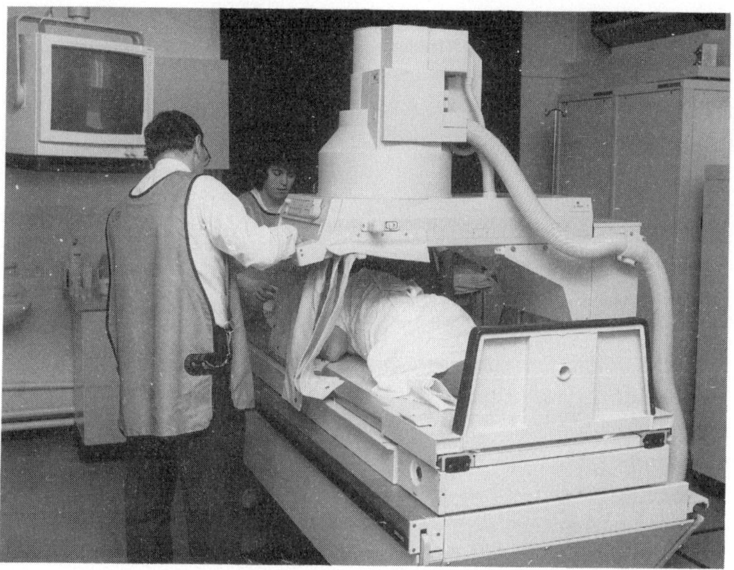

Fig. 3.1 Fluoroscopic screening in progress.

Patient acceptability. Figure 3.1 shows a screening room in use. The apparatus can be a little threatening, particularly for claustrophobic patients and children, but this is seldom a problem given some explanation and reassurance. The X-ray tube is usually under the table, and the image intensifier is suspended over the patient, and brought as close as possible to the body surface during screening. The table can be tilted through at least ninety degrees, and the table top moves horizontally in two or four directions. This can all be a little disorientating, especially for elderly patients.

Digital subtraction angiography (DSA)

Initially known as digital vascular imaging (DVI), this is a refinement of the screening technique described in the previous section. It is most often used in angiographic examinations, the fluoroscopic images obtained before and after contrast injection being stored in digital form. The initial frames can then be electronically subtracted from later images, the difference image so formed showing the contrast-filled vessels unobscured by other structures. This permits the use of lower doses of contrast medium, or by injecting large volumes of contrast into a central vein, it is sometimes possible to avoid arterial catheterization altogether.

Computed tomography (CT scanning)

Since its arrival on the scene in the early seventies, CT scanning has developed rapidly, and the hardware has become cheaper, smaller, and easier to operate. It is now possible to house a modern compact machine in a normal sized radiographic room.

The patient lies at the centre of rotation of a circular gantry on one side of which is a radiation detector, and on the other, the X-ray tube. The beam of radiation passes through the patient, and the degree of attenuation of the beam by the patient's tissues is recorded as a number. Tube and detector then rotate around the patient in small steps, repeating the measurement many times over. The computer is then able to deduce the internal structure of the body in the plane of the gantry, displaying the result on a monitor as a 'slice' through the patient. Table and patient advance through the gantry and a series of such slices is built up.

The role of CT. CT has found a place in almost every area of diagnostic radiology, and later chapters document its role in specific situations. Appropriately used, CT can often provide a short cut to the diagnosis, but it is relatively expensive, and scanning time is at a premium in most hospitals. Consequently, vetting of requests by the responsible radiologist is necessary to ensure that the technique is only used in those cases where it is likely to be useful.

Patient acceptability. Claustrophobia can be a problem (Fig. 3.2), although this is more often seen with MRI (below). The patient having an abdominal scan may be required to drink some dilute contrast medium, or to have contrast or air administered rectally if the pelvic contents are being examined. Sometimes intravenous contrast is used, as for an IVU (see Chapter 4).

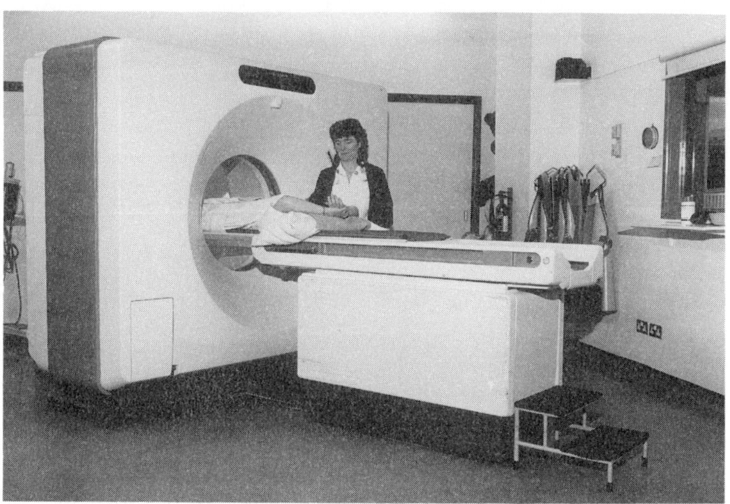

Fig. 3.2 Computed tomography (CT) scanner in use.

Nuclear medicine (NM)

The only similarity between nuclear medicine and what has gone before is the use of ionizing radiation. NM gives much more information about the function of an organ or system than the other imaging methods. The inevitable trade-off comes in its inferior spatial resolution. For this reason, NM is often used as a complement to other methods, but there will be many occasions where you are not really interested in anatomical detail, and the isotope study will be all you need.

The steps involved in performing a nuclear medicine study are outlined in Table 3.1. The isotope most frequently used is technetium 99m (^{99}mTc). This combines a suitably short half-life of six hours with chemical reactivity, allowing the easy labelling of a large number of different radiopharmaceuticals. It is also readily available in the form of a generator which contains the parent radionuclide; this decays continuously into ^{99}mTc which can be milked off as required. A generator lasts for about a week.

Table 3.1　Stages in the performance of an isotope scan

1. Select isotope—usually ^{99}Tc, but others are used (e.g. thallium, gallium)
2. Choose a pharmaceutical which will be taken up in, or processed by, the organ under investigation
3. Label the pharmaceutical *in vitro* with the isotope
4. Inject the labelled pharmaceutical intravenously
5. If necessary, wait for the pharmaceutical to be taken up by the target organ/tissue
6. Start acquiring images

The image is formed by the gamma camera (Fig. 3.3). This contains an array of radiation detectors which map the emitted radiation and store the result digitally until required for processing. Thus it is possible to acquire multiple images very quickly over short periods of time. This ability to perform 'dynamic' imaging means that we are able to follow the passage of a radiopharmaceutical through the body, and so measure function in addition to acquiring static images of an organ.

Patient acceptability. Nearly as good as ultrasound (see below). An intravenous injection is required, but unlike radiographic

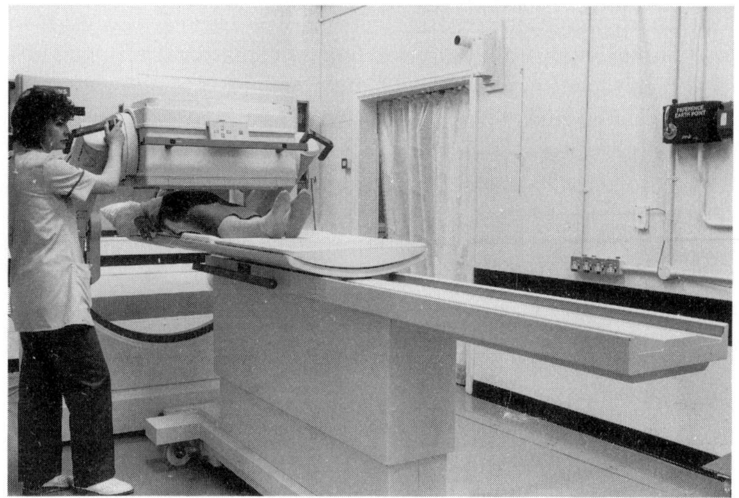

Fig. 3.3 Gamma camera in use.

contrast media (Chapter 2), adverse reactions to radiopharmaceuticals are very rare. Most NM investigations require little or no preparation.

Imaging without ionizing radiation

Ultrasound

The advent of modern, high quality, real-time ultrasound has probably been the greatest single advance in imaging in the last twenty years, and almost certainly the most cost-effective. It avoids the use of ionizing radiation, relying instead on the detection of reflected high-frequency sound waves.

The ultrasound probe, or transducer, sends a beam of sound into the tissues, the waves being emitted in small pulses lasting a microsecond or so. A thousand of these pulses are emitted per second, and so the transducer is only acting as a transmitter for one thousandth of the time. Between pulses, it acts as a receiver, picking up the reflected sound waves and reconstructing them into a two dimensional monitor image. This picture is updated many times per second, giving a moving (real-time) image on the monitor. The image can be frozen at any time and hard copy made; alternatively, the examination can be recorded on video-tape.

Transducer design has advanced rapidly, and in addition to the standard body surface probes, there are models designed for rectal, vaginal, endoscopic and intra-operative use. Machines are mobile, and can be taken into the ward, intensive care unit or operating theatre.

Patient acceptability. Ultrasound is just about ideal from the patient's point of view. It is painless and non-invasive, and even for the most claustrophobic patient, the machinery is non-threatening (Fig. 3.4).

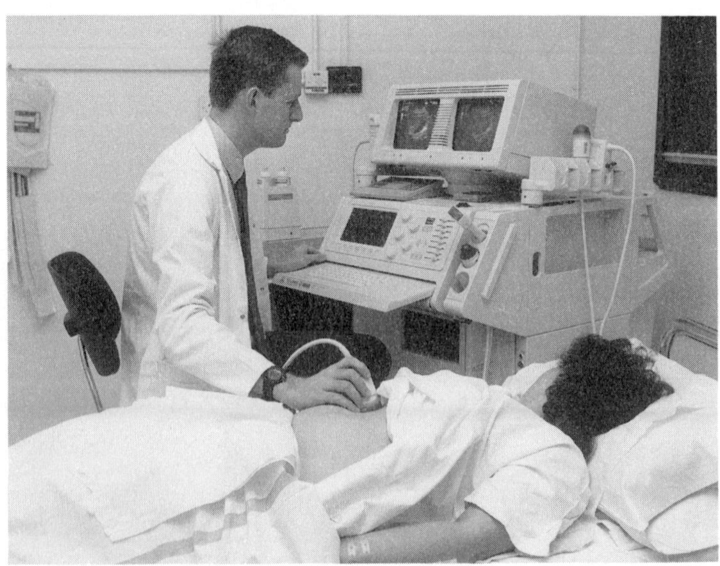

Fig. 3.4 An ultrasound scan in progress.

Limitations of ultrasound. The physics of ultrasound mean that the quality of the image is dependent on patient physique to a greater extent than is the case for some other techniques. The sound beam is scattered and distorted by gas (e.g. in bowel or lung) and attenuated by fat. Generally speaking, better results are obtained in thin patients than fat, and bowel gas may obscure deep organs such as the pancreas, no matter how skilled the operator. Luckily, in CT, gas is not a problem, and fat is a positive advantage is separating adjacent viscera. Thus CT is a useful alternative in patients where good quality ultrasound images cannot be obtained.

Doppler ultrasound

This is simply a different way of using ultrasound, and most modern machines incorporate a Doppler option. It relies on the fact that if the ultrasound beam is reflected by a moving structure, such as a column of blood in a vessel, there will be a difference between the transmitted and received frequency—a Doppler shift. By analysing this shift, it is possible to extract information about flow velocity, and even to colour-code the output so that flow in vessels is demonstrated in real-time, different colours indicating different directions of flow.

The value of Doppler scanning is now well-established in echocardiography and vascular work in general. As machines become more widely available its role is likely to be extended.

Magnetic resonance imaging (MRI)

Originally known as nuclear magnetic resonance (NMR) scanning, this is the latest development in imaging technology, and its role is still being defined.

MRI relies on the fact that the body contains lots of hydrogen nuclei, each of them acting as a magnetic dipole. If the body is subjected to a strong, uniform, magnetic field, these nuclei align with it like small magnets. If a radiofrequency (RF) signal pulse is applied, the nuclei transiently alter their axis and then return to their original state, in the process emitting their own RF signal. By a clever manipulation of the field gradients, a cross-sectional image of the body can be built up. The pictures look similar to those produced by a CT scanner, but no ionizing radiation is used, and sections can be obtained in any plane. By using different pulse sequences, different types of information can be obtained concerning the tissues.

Areas where it is already clear that MRI has a lot to offer are imaging of the CNS and musculoskeletal system, including the spine: it may well replace radiculography and arthrography, for example. Cost is likely to limit availability in the UK for the immediate future, and for this reason, tight vetting of requests will be necessary.

Patient acceptability. As for CT, but the problems for claustrophobic patients are worse, due to the tunnel-like configuration of the gantry, although the latest generation of machines is less intimidating than earlier models.

4

The patient's view

In this chapter we shall cover a few commonly requested procedures which make significant demands on the patient, either because of the actual mechanics of the investigation, or in the preparation required. All too frequently patients attend the radiology department with no idea of what awaits them, or the reasons for the planned investigation. It is not good medical practice to refer a patient for a barium enema with the words 'I'm just sending you up to the hospital for an X-ray of your bowel', and yet it happens all too often. Hopefully this chapter, and the remainder of the book, will give you the information you need to prepare the patient mentally for their examination (see p. 7). Chapter three includes some general points on the patient acceptability of the newer imaging techniques, and brief details of all the other investigations you are likely to request will be found in the glossary (p. 134).

Barium swallow and meal

Preparation

Barium meals are scheduled for a morning screening list wherever possible, in which case the patient will be asked to fast from midnight. In the case of an afternoon appointment, they will be allowed an early light breakfast. If the patient is a diabetic, we try to give them the first appointment of the day, and arrange for them to eat immediately after the examination.

On the day

After undressing and putting on a gown, the patient is taken into the screening room where the radiographer and/or radiologist will explain the procedure. At some stage, not necessarily the beginning, the radiologist will administer an intravenous injection of either glucagon or Buscopan to reduce gastrointestinal motility, and ask the patient to swallow some effervescent tablets or granules. The fizzy tablets and the injection are part of the double contrast technique which is now routine in most departments, the intention being to leave the stomach and duodenum distended by gas with a thin layer of barium coating the mucosa (Fig. 4.1).

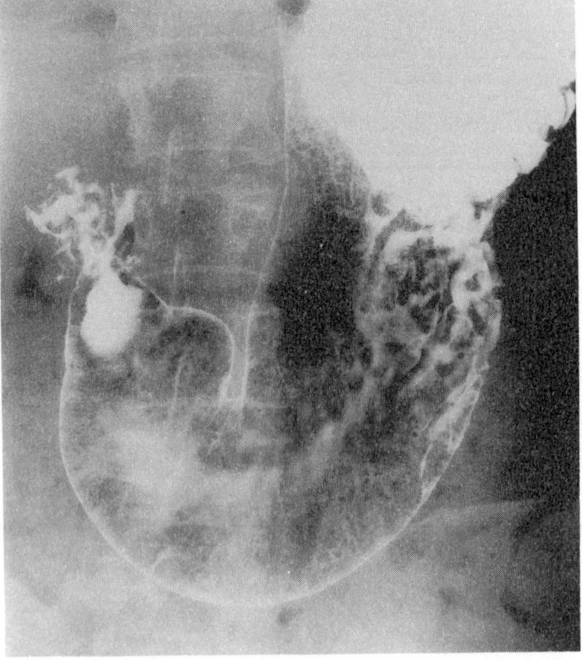

Fig. 4.1 One frame from a double contrast barium meal showing the stomach distended with gas and a thin layer of barium coating the mucosa.

The patient is then taken to the screening table (see Chapter 3, p. 21), usually starting in the upright position, and begins to drink the barium. During screening, films will be taken and cine or video recording may be used for the swallow. A considerable amount of rolling around and movement of the table is required to demonstrate all parts of the upper GIT in double contrast, and this is too much for some frail or sick patients. In this case, the technique may need to be modified. This may limit the diagnostic value of the procedure, and endoscopy will often be the chosen procedure in these patients.

After-effects

Usually none, but elderly patients may be upset by all the rolling around, particularly if Buscopan has been used. They should therefore be advised to bring a friend or relative with them. The barium can have a constipating effect, again particularly in the elderly, and they will be advised to drink plenty of fluids on returning home.

Fit patients will be able to drive themselves home, although in the rare event of the Buscopan affecting their vision, they may need to wait in the department for 20 minutes or so until the effects wear off.

Barium enema

Preparation

A clean colon is essential for the double contrast technique which most radiologists now use, and details of the preparation will vary between hospitals. Most protocols prescribe a low-residue diet for 24 or 48 hours prior to the appointment, with fluids only on the day. This is accompanied by a saline purgative given in two doses on the day before the enema, or a single dose of a senna preparation. Some departments still use a colonic washout immediately before the enema, but this practice is becoming less widespread. The routine will be modified for some patients, for example those with inflammatory bowel disease. Details will be given in the relevant chapters.

On the day

The patient will lie on the screening table either prone or in the left lateral position. The nozzle of the enema tube is inserted by either the nurse or the radiologist, and barium runs in under screening control from a bag suspended over the table. Once the barium column is beyond the hepatic flexure, air is insufflated to push the barium round to the caecum and distend the colon. The end result is a gas-distended colon with a thin layer of barium coating the mucosa (Fig. 4.2), allowing the detection of small

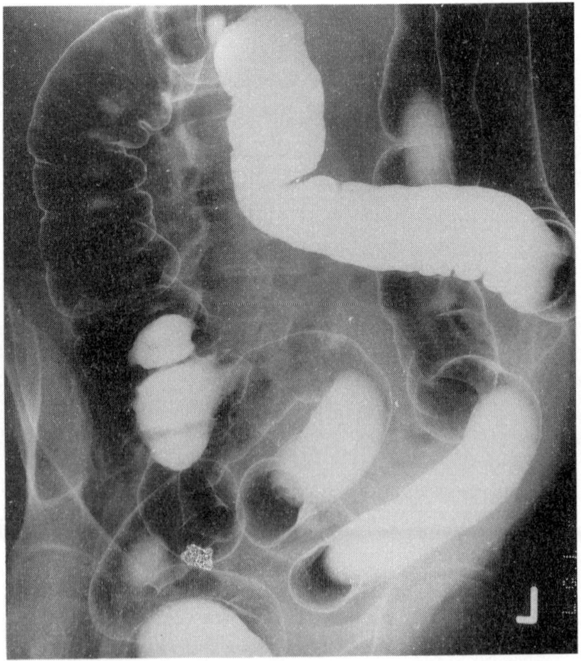

Fig. 4.2   One view from a barium enema examination, again showing double contrast effect.

lesions such as polyps—hence the need for a clean mucosa. Intravenous glucagon or Buscopan may be used routinely, or just in those patients where spasm is a problem. Films are taken with the patient in various positions to ensure that all parts of the colon are seen in double contrast. When they have been checked by the radiologist, the patient will be allowed to go to the toilet and evacuate the barium. Another picture may be taken after this. The whole procedure takes around forty minutes (more if a preliminary washout is used).

After-effects

No matter how gentle and sympathetic the radiologist and radiographer might be, a barium enema is an uncomfortable and undignified procedure for the patient. Some will have difficulty retaining the barium and will feel thoroughly humiliated.

Elderly patients should be accompanied by a friend or relative wherever possible, as they can feel fairly exhausted by the end of the examination, and they may also be upset by the rigorous purgation used in the preparation. Younger patients will have fewer problems, but they will still not enjoy the experience.

Intravenous urogram (IVU)

Preparation

It used to be common practice to dehydrate patients for up to 12 hours prior to urography. The aim was to ensure maximum concentration of the contrast medium in the collecting system of the kidney. With the higher doses of contrast medium now used routinely, this is no longer necessary, and in some patients it can be positively dangerous (see Chapter 2). Most preparation regimes still include the instruction to take nil by mouth for at least four hours, but this is chiefly to reduce the risk of vomiting in response to the contrast injection. Patients will usually be given a purgative to help clear the colon of solid faeces which can mask the renal areas.

On the day

After a plain abdominal radiograph to detect any calcification, the radiographer and/or the radiologist will question the patient about any history of allergy or previous contrast reaction before giving the injection into a vein. During and immediately after the injection, most patients experience a feeling of warmth and an odd taste. Nausea is fairly common, and an unfortunate minority vomit.

The radiographer then takes a series of radiographs, the exact sequence depending on the clinical information required. Compression may be applied using an abdominal binder in order to obtain maximal distension of the renal pelvis: this is uncomfortable. The examination usually ends with a post-micturition film, and normally takes less than an hour, unless delayed films are required in a patient with obstructed kidneys.

After-effects

Hopefully none, but see Chapter two for a discussion of contrast medium reactions.

Ultrasound

The basic principles of ultrasound are explained in Chapter three, but a few additional points are worth mentioning here.

Preparation

Patients are often confused by the word 'scan', and turn up expecting to be 'put into a big machine'. A few words of explanation at the time of the decision to refer can help to allay any anxiety. Physical preparation will depend on the area of the abdomen being examined. For upper abdominal scans patients will be fasted in order to minimize the amount of gas present and to ensure that the gallbladder is full. For pelvic scanning, they must have a full bladder—this acts as a window on to the pelvic viscera.

You must therefore be explicit in your referrals—do not ask for 'abdominal ultrasound' if you are interested in the pelvis. If you want the abdomen and pelvis looking at, we will give the patient water to fill the bladder and fast them to avoid gallbladder stimulation. Remember that milk is a food, and a potent stimulator of gallbladder emptying.

In some female patients it is difficult to achieve adequate bladder filling. Ultrasound using a transvaginal probe can be useful here, as a full bladder is not required. Transvaginal scanning will also be used as a routine for some gynaecological examinations (e.g. monitoring follicle development in infertility).

5

Heart and lungs

Some topics will be covered in the vascular section and others, for example specialized cardiovascular investigations, will be outside the scope of this book. We hope we have included all of the commonly encountered problems where imaging has a part to play.

Emergency imaging

Acute dyspnoea—? cause

The CXR is the only initial imaging investigation likely to aid management, but it may not be diagnostic and must be taken in conjunction with the clinical findings.

For example, the chest X-ray (CXR) of a patient that you suspect is in heart failure may show typical radiographic features. All too often, however, it reveals a largish heart with some patchy consolidation (see glossary of terms) that could be due to oedema, infection, or both. The X-ray beam cannot distinguish between oedema, pus, blood, inhaled beer, or even solid tumour. The differentiation between these different pathologies can often be made from associated radiographic features which can be very subtle, so get the film reported ASAP!

Serial examinations (at sensible intervals) often give a better indication of the underlying problem than a single radiograph which is a snapshot of a disease process which may progress for months or years.

Chest pain—? myocardial infarction (MI)
(also see the section on cold imaging, p. 39)

This question is frequently seen on CXR request forms. There are no specific radiographic features of MI, and the main purpose of the examination is to exclude other causes of chest pain (e.g. pneumonia). Many patients die from myocardial infarction with a normal CXR.

The diagnosis is usually made on the basis of clinical findings, ECG changes, and enzyme levels. The only other imaging technique which may be helpful in difficult cases is scintigraphy using thallium, pyrophosphate or, more recently, radiolabelled antimyosin. Timing is critical if these techniques are to give a meaningful result, so consult your radiologist/nuclear medicine physician, or follow the established protocol if one exists.

Suspected pneumothorax

The CXR is the only imaging test required. Small pneumothoraces are sometimes better demonstrated on an expiratory film. You may have to inspect the film very closely to see small apical pneumothoraces, but these are of doubtful clinical significance.

If the films show evidence of a tension pneumothorax, the radiologist will usually inform you so that prompt action can be taken. If there is no radiological opinion immediately available, mediastinal shift away from the side of the pneumothorax should alert you to the possibility of tension.

Follow-up films should be spaced sensibly, and an expiratory film will normally be sufficient, there is no need to routinely obtain two films.

Dissection of the thoracic aorta
See vascular section, p. 105.

Suspected pulmonary embolus (PE)

The CXR will be the first investigation. It is seldom possible to make a diagnosis of PE from the chest film alone, which may frequently be normal. If embolus proceeds to infarction (and most do not), then the resulting patch of consolidation will be indistinguishable from that due to infection. The mainstay of diagnosis of PE is the isotope lung scan.

Lung (V/O or V/P) scan. Ventilation is assessed using radio-active gas or aerosol, and a map of pulmonary perfusion is obtained by the intravenous injection of tiny labelled protein particles which become trapped in the lung capillary bed. A typical embolus produces perfusion defects in areas of lung which are normally ventilated. Studies correlating different scan patterns with the findings of pulmonary angiography allow us to assess the probability that a particular patient has suffered a PE on the basis of their scan result. The report you receive will assign the patient to one of the following groups on the basis of the scan appearance:

1. *Normal.* The most useful result—it effectively excludes PE as the cause of the patient's symptoms.

2. *Low probability of PE.* This is not the same as a normal result: the scan is abnormal, but the probability of embolus is 10–15 per cent at most.

3. *Intermediate probability.* The likelihood of PE in patients in this group may be as low as 30 per cent or as high as 70 per cent depending on the pattern of abnormalities.

4. *High probability.* Classical unmatched perfusion defects— the likelihood of them being embolic is 90 per cent plus.

The scan result is just one more piece of information to be weighed in balance with the clinical findings, ECG result, blood gases etc. Even an intermediate probability result is useful: it tells you that PE cannot be excluded, and will often be enough, in conjunction with other findings, to allow you to go ahead with treatment. Your chances of an unequivocal result are increased if you ask for the scan as soon as the diagnosis of PE is considered, and hopefully while the CXR is still normal. However, many of these patients have chronic lung disease, and the scan appearance will be non-specific.

Remember that a recent CXR (preferably within 12 hours of the scan) must be available in order to interpret the scan.

Pulmonary arteriography is widely regarded as the gold standard in the diagnosis of PE, but it is not widely practised for several reasons. It is invasive, and selective catheterization of subdivisions of the main pulmonary arteries may be required if accurate results are to be obtained. In some series up to 20 per cent of patients are considered unfit for such a prolonged study. However, angiography may be required in patients with an equivocal scan result where anticoagulant treatment is likely to be particularly hazardous. It will also be performed prior to embolectomy or thrombolytic therapy.

Acute asthma

The diagnosis is usually made on the basis of clinical findings and lung function tests, and frequently the patient will have a long history of recurrent problems. The CXR is often normal, and its main use is in identifying complications such as pneumothorax or cardiac failure. See also the section on cardiac failure below.

'Cold' imaging

Chest pain/angina

Chest pain presenting as an emergency is covered above.

Patients with less acute symptoms will have had a CXR, and you need to think carefully before requesting further imaging procedures. The diagnosis of ischaemic heart disease (IHD) will usually be made on clinical, ECG, and biochemical findings, the CXR being useful in excluding some other causes of pain.

If suspicion of IHD persists, and all other tests have been equivocal, nuclear cardiology has an important role to play. A thallium scan will be indicated, and is particularly useful in deciding which patients need to go on to coronary angiography. Echocardiography also has a role here. It will identify regional wall motion abnormalities, and also give an estimate of the ejection fraction. As we said in Chapter one, there is no point asking for these additional imaging procedures in patients whose pre-test probability of IHD is already high on purely clinical grounds.

Remember that chest pain can be due to oesophageal disease (see p. 52).

Hypertension

A common presenting problem. Invariably, the patient will have a CXR, although it seldom makes much contribution to management in patients whose only clinical problem is their high blood pressure. There is certainly no indication for regular repeat films at every outpatient review. The contribution of imaging in patients whose hypertension is thought to be due to renovascular disease is outlined in Chapter 7 (p. 68).

Cardiac failure

This is covered in the section on acute dyspnoea (above), but not all patients present acutely. Again, we emphasize the limited role of the CXR. We receive a lot of requests for CXRs in ambulant outpatients, giving the clinical history as 'CCF ? degree of failure'. Most of these are inappropriate requests originating at spinal level—you will make your treatment decisions on clinical grounds, not on the CXR appearance.

Heart murmur/suspected valvular disease/septal defect

Although it is often possible to suggest the presence of a specific valvular problem on the CXR appearance alone, the diagnosis of murmurs has traditionally been the province of the physician and his or her stethoscope, with cardiac catheterization as the invasive gold standard. With the advent of echocardiography it has become possible to quantify non-invasively the degree of valvular stenosis/regurgitation or the degree of shunting in the case of a septal defect. Scintigraphy can also be useful in quantifying shunts.

Acute chest infection

The CXR is useful in the initial diagnosis. Follow-up should be clinical, unless or until there are signs of complications or delay in resolution. At least one follow-up film is sensible in the middle aged or elderly patient, particularly if they are smokers.

Haemoptysis

Most patients with haemoptysis will have a CXR which is either normal or non-specifically abnormal. Although a CXR is justifiable, the patient with a convincing history will require bronchoscopy whatever the result of the radiograph, either to demonstrate an endobronchial lesion not seen on the CXR, or to obtain cells from a radiographically visible lesion. Although CT is a superior technique for showing lung tumours (see below), it is not feasible to use it on all patients whose symptoms might be due to neoplasm.

Chronic lung disease

A common clinical problem, which generates far more chest radiography than it need. The CXR shows gross morphological change, but gives much less physiological information (which is what really matters) than the lung function tests, in particular, the blood gases and transfer factor. Although the CXR is of little use in monitoring the progress of the chronic lung disease itself, it will of course, be indicated if you suspect the patient has developed complications, such as acute pneumonia or neoplasm.

Lung tumour

We are considering here the situation where a presumed tumour has been revealed on a CXR performed either for non-specific symptoms or for respiratory tract problems. Occasionally tumours are demonstrated unexpectedly on a radiograph taken for some other purpose. Once a possible tumour has been diagnosed, there is little to be gained from further plain films, although the radiologist will sometimes ask for other views or even standard tomography just to confirm that a lesion is genuine.

The definitive examination is bronchoscopy to obtain cytological proof of the diagnosis, followed by CT to stage the tumour if it is confirmed to be malignant. Plain radiography is very poor at demonstrating mediastinal disease (see below) and cannot therefore be used to assess resectability. For some peripheral tumours, CT with percutaneous biopsy will be preferable to bronchoscopy. Under scanning control fine needles can be directed very accurately, avoiding major vessels and other vulnerable structures. Some lesions can be biopsied percutaneously under ordinary X-ray screening control if CT is not readily available.

Metastatic disease

It is now accepted that CT is more sensitive in detecting metastases than the CXR, and in the staging and follow-up of tumours where lung metastases are common and have implications for treatment (e.g. testicular tumours), CT scanning will usually be incorporated into the protocol. Similarly, CT will be indicated when the CXR has shown a mass that could be a metastasis, and you want to see if there are others present which were not revealed on the plain film.

Mediastinal disease

As mentioned in the previous section, the CXR may be relatively normal in the presence of extensive mediastinal disease, and so the accurate diagnosis and monitoring of mediastinal lymph-adenopathy or other pathology requires CT scanning. This doesn't mean that all patients with mediastinal disease require repeated CT scans. For example, interval CXRs are perfectly adequate to monitor the resolution of lymphadenopathy in a patient who presents with sarcoidosis and who is responding well to treatment. With lymphoma or other malignancy where knowledge of disease extent and response is crucial to management, CT will be necessary. The relative roles of CT and MRI are still being worked out.

Thoracic cage abnormalities

Rib fractures will be dealt with in the section on trauma (p. 112). Focal non-traumatic thoracic cage lesions can be demonstrated on the CXR, but remember that CXR exposures are optimized for the heart, lungs, and mediastinum, and not for bone. If it is likely to aid patient management, specific rib views should be requested.

Assessment of costo-vertebral disease and demonstration of the sternum are very difficult with plain radiography, and when pathology in either of these areas is suspected, CT will usually be the answer.

Just occasionally, if there is a strong suspicion of a rib lesion and radiography is normal, scintigraphy will be indicated to confirm or exclude the presence of active bone pathology.

The CXR in non-specific illness

As mentioned in previous sections, the CXR is frequently requested in patients with non-specific symptoms such as malaise and weight loss. This is perfectly reasonable—we have all seen patients (from other hospitals, of course!) whose pulmonary TB was only picked-up when a CXR was finally requested after numerous other investigations.

Requests to avoid!

1. *Pre-op chest please*

Routine radiography of patients of any age prior to non-cardiopulmonary surgery has been shown to be of no value, and the practice has now hopefully been discontinued in most centres. CXR is only recommended in the following instances:

1) patients with chest symptoms;
2) patients with a known primary malignancy (to look for metastases);
3) patients from ethnic groups with a high incidence of TB and who have not had a CXR in the preceding 6 months.

Please note: these are not 'routine' CXRs, they are being performed for a purpose, and the relevant clinical information should be given on the request form.

2. *'Screening CXR'*

For example for malignancy, pre-employment, on admission to hospital etc. Sadly, even 6 monthly CXRs in a high risk population have been shown to have no effect on the survival rate from bronchial carcinoma. Similarly, so-called routine radiography of asymptomatic populations for whatever purpose is a waste of resources.

6

Gastrointestinal tract

Emergency imaging

Acute non-specific abdominal pain

The erect chest X-ray is useful to show free gas under the diaphragm in cases of gastrointestinal perforation and may also reveal abnormalities above the diaphragm which can sometimes present as abdominal pain.

A supine abdominal radiograph may show evidence of bowel disease (e.g. obstruction, perforation, acute inflammation) or calcification. (See specific pathologies below.)

A variety of calcifications may be demonstrated—gall stones, renal calculi, and appendicoliths. Beware not to over-diagnose, as insignificant calcifications (mesenteric glands, pelvic phleboliths etc.) are common. Calcification within aortic aneurysms may be evident, but will not help you decide if the aneurysm is the source of the current symptoms.

Occasionally, enlargement of specific abdominal viscera can be diagnosed, but cross sectional imaging (e.g. ultrasound or CT) is required to confirm the finding. Beware!! Soft tissue masses can be simulated by normal structures—particularly fluid filled bowel.

Now what? You really need to decide upon the most likely diagnosis or diagnoses from the clinical presentation, physical examination, and plain radiographic findings, and direct your investigations accordingly. For example, a useful division is between bowel and the rest of the abdominal viscera as the latter can be investigated by ultrasound, whereas bowel, with a few exceptions, cannot. See the following sections for investigation of specific diagnoses.

Mallory–Weiss

This is best investigated with endoscopy as it not only demonstrates the mucosal tear, but can also say whether active bleeding is occurring.

Acute dysphagia

Endoscopy or a contrast examination are both suitable. Low density barium or a non-ionic contrast medium is used for a contrast examination, in order to minimize any pulmonary damage if the patient aspirates. Gastrografin is not suitable due to its severe irritant effect on the lungs.

Acute peptic ulcer disease

Perforation. AXR and CXR (as above) to look for free gas (it may of course not be due to perforation of an ulcer). If the patient is not able to stand for a CXR, a horizontal beam abdominal film with the patient lying on their left side is an alternative way to demonstrate free gas. Localized leak into lesser sac etc. can be demonstrated with oral contrast but seldom affects management.

Acute pain. Ulcers can be demonstrated by barium meal or endoscopy. If there is evidence of gastric out-flow obstruction, gastric intubation and aspiration must be performed before either examination. Presence of fluid or food within the stomach hampers views of the mucosa on endoscopy and prevents adequate barium coating of the gastric mucosa during double contrast barium examination.

Acute gastrointestinal bleeding

(a) Haematemesis. Endoscopy is indicated as it can determine not only the presence of any pathology but also ascertain if the lesion has recently bled. Barium meal is less suitable as a first line investigation unless endoscopy is not available.

(b) Profuse rectal bleeding. Direct inspection at least of the rectum and sigmoid should be performed. This will exclude obvious low colonic sources of bleeding without the necessity to implement more complex imaging investigations. If the patient's condition allows, colonscopy may be possible. Often the presence of large quantities of blood within the bowel prevents observation of the bleeding point. Barium examinations of the large bowel are inappropriate as prompt identification of the bleeding source is required.

If either haematemesis or profuse rectal bleeding continue undiagnosed, scintigraphy or arteriography, or both, may be employed. Scintigraphy is probably more sensitive and certainly less invasive than angiography, but does not localize the bleeding point so accurately. For angiographic localization the patient needs to be bleeding at the time of the examination, but scintigraphy with labelled RBCs (see glossary of investigations) will allow imaging for up to 24 hours and can therefore be useful in intermittent bleeding (see also below). Consult your radiologist.

Bowel obstruction

Supine abdominal X-ray is normally all that is required. Erect or decubitus (see glossary of terms) abdominal views are useful to demonstrate confirmatory signs (such as air/fluid levels), but are not strictly necessary and do not help differentiate between obstruction and ileus. The only feature which may be helpful in this respect is localized bowel dilatation, which is more likely to be due to a mechanical cause than to ileus. The level of obstruction may be deduced from the pattern of gaseous bowel distension, and the configuration of the distended viscus may be useful in diagnosing volvulus. Gas overlying or below the pelvic rami may indicate the presence of a hernia.

Low colonic (descending colon, sigmoid colon, and rectum) obstruction with an incompetent ileo–caecal valve may produce dilatation of all levels of large and small bowel. Thus large bowel obstruction can mimic global ileus.

Occasionally, dilated bowel may be fluid filled and therefore not evident on plain radiographs other than as an amorphous greyness and absence of normal gas pattern. Ultrasound can be useful in these cases.

Water soluble contrast enema. This can be used to confirm the presence of true colonic obstruction. The examination merely aims to show the presence or absence of an obstructing lesion, and in the unprepared bowel is unlikely to give a definitive diagnosis of the pathology concerned. For technical reasons, it is much less accurate in diagnosing obstructing lesions of the right colon.

Acute inflammatory bowel disease—see also cold imaging section (below)

In the context of acute imaging this usually means acute colitis. A plain abdominal film may show thickened bowel wall and occasionally mucosal polyps. Toxic dilatation of the colon is present if the diameter of the transverse colon exceeds 5.5 cm. This is a very important finding. If bowel necrosis has occurred gas may be seen within the bowel wall or even occasionally in portal veins. An 'instant enema', a gentle barium enema (without bowel preparation) may be used to assess the extent and severity of disease if early surgical intervention is contemplated. *This must not be performed* if there is any suspicion of toxic dilatation.

In some centres gastroenterologists assess the presence and severity of disease with flexible sigmoidoscopy and/or colono-scopy. The major risks relate to perforation in the acute phase and colonoscopy, with its need for insufflation, should be avoided if there is any suspicion of toxic dilatation.

Acute appendicitis

The diagnosis is usually made on clinical grounds. The AXR may show localized ileus or a calcified appendicolith, but often the changes are non-specific and unhelpful. Useful primary investigation if clinical diagnosis is unclear. Ultrasound is useful in children (see Chapter 14, p. 24), but is less so in adults. It may be used in the demonstration of the complications of acute appendicitis such as abscess formation. Barium studies are not indicated.

Acute cholecystitis

Ultrasound is the primary investigation method of all biliary disease including acute cholecystitis. It may show calculi, wall thickening, and most usefully focal tenderness of the gall bladder which may not be apparent on clinical examination.

If ultrasound is negative or inconclusive but there is still a strong clinical suspicion of cholecystitis, the next investigation is a HIDA scan, particularly if your surgeons operate on 'hot' gallbladders.

Oral cholecystogram is less sensitive and less accurate than ultrasound and is not indicated.

Biliary colic

An abdominal X-ray can be useful to detect radiopaque calculi and the presence of gas within bile ducts, but ultrasound is the primary investigation method. It is extremely accurate in the detection of gallbladder stones but less so in the detection of duct calculi, which are often obscured by gas in the duodenum. The presence of CBD dilatation (in the absence of previous surgery) is a good indicator of acute biliary pathology. The gold standard investigation for biliary duct calculi is ERCP. In acute biliary colic with evidence of biliary obstruction, ERCP can be combined with therapeutic sphincterotomy.

Jaundice ? cause

Ultrasound is the primary investigation method for jaundice and will distinguish between obstructive and non-obstructive jaundice by demonstrating the presence or absence of dilated bile ducts. One major proviso is that ducts may take a little time to dilate and therefore an ultrasound scan performed too early may show normal calibre ducts. Pre-existing parenchymal liver disease may also prevent dilatation of intrahepatic ducts.

Ultrasound will usually indicate the level of any obstruction, but is not so good at demonstrating the cause. In particular, problems occur with lower CBD calculi, cholangiocarcinomas, and small peri-ampullary lesions of the pancreas; it will however demonstrate a proportion of duct calculi and the larger obstructing tumours. If obstructive jaundice is diagnosed and the cause or site remain unclear, a direct contrast cholangiogram is required. This is usually performed by ERCP which has the added advantage of directly visualizing the ampulla. When ERCP is impossible (e.g. previous gastric surgery with Roux-en-Y configuration), direct cholangiography via PTC (see glossary, p. 136) is performed. In malignant obstruction, CT or MRI may be employed to give further information concerning the extent of disease. Some tumours (e.g. cholangiocarcinoma) have distinctive appearances on CT but biopsy (ultrasound or CT guided) is usually required for a definitive diagnosis.

See pp. 146 and 148 for further discussion of interventional biliary procedures.

Cholangitis

Abdominal X-ray may show gas within the biliary tree. This may also be present if a gallstone has eroded into the bowel or a sphincterotomy has been performed. Ultrasound is more sensitive in the demonstration of gas, and may show non-specific inflammatory changes in the liver and/or liver abscess formation. The diagnosis is usually made by a combination of clinical, microbiological, and imaging evidence.

Acute pancreatitis

The diagnosis is made on clinical and biochemical grounds and imaging has two roles. First, to detect the complications of pancreatitis, particularly pancreatic necrosis and secondary fluid collections, and second, to detect the cause, especially gallstones.

Early ultrasound scanning is often unproductive due to the presence of gastrointestinal ileus, which masks the pancreas at a time in the patient's illness when oral fluids cannot be given to aid an ultrasound examination. After a delay of 4–5 days the examination has much greater diagnostic yield and usually gallstones can be confidently proven or excluded.

CT is the definitive examination of the acutely inflamed pancreas and, with dynamic contrast-enhanced techniques, can accurately map necrotic and viable areas of pancreas. It is also the best technique available for demonstrating the size and location of pancreatic fluid collections, which can often be managed satisfactorily by percutaneous drainage with CT or ultrasound guidance.

In some patients with fulminating acute pancreatitis the acute phase may last for a considerable length of time. Imaging during this period is usually aimed at the diagnosis and monitoring of complications, particularly necrosis and fluid collections. Frequently, repeat CT scans are performed within short intervals with a considerable radiation dose to the patient. It is likely that when MRI becomes more widely available this will be used instead of CT.

Trauma

See section on non-skeletal trauma, Chapter 13.

'Cold imaging'

Dysphagia

Barium swallow, either recorded as a video or fast sequence radiographs, gives a good view of the dynamics of swallowing and any lesion that might be present. Endoscopy is the second line investigation aimed at determining the nature of any pathology identified.

Oesophageal pain—'heartburn', or 'atypical chest pain'

Oesophageal pain is a great mimic, but once clinical suspicion has been aroused, the imaging should proceed as follows: Barium swallow is the first line investigation. As described above, fast sequence imaging gives an overview of the dynamics of oesophageal motility and the examination may demonstrate gastro-oesophageal reflux with or without associated mucosal changes of oesophagitis. Endoscopy cannot demonstrate motility disorders but is better at visualizing the mucosal changes of oesophagitis, and of course, biopsy is possible. Scintigraphy is used in some centres to demonstrate gastro-oesophageal reflux and it is claimed that this is a more physiological examination than barium studies. It is certainly a useful alternative to oesophageal manometry and pH measurement in oesophageal motility disorders.

Dyspepsia

Endoscopy or barium meal can be used. Both have false negative rates but can be highly dependable in expert hands. Endoscopy permits biopsy and barium meal gives a better overview of the upper gastrointestinal tract and better illustrates features such as gastro-oesophageal reflux and gastric emptying.

Endoscopy needs sedation in most patients and is not well tolerated by all. Barium meal is a rigorous examination involving rolling the patient on the hard table to coat the stomach mucosa and is not suitable for the infirm. The request 'barium meal please—patient not fit for endoscopy' is frequently seen and makes no sense.

Barium meal (or endoscopy), may not be indicated in all dyspeptic patients. Older patients with dyspepsia, anorexia, and weight loss undoubtedly need investigation, but younger dyspeptic patients are frequently given a trial of H_2 antagonists before specific investigation is undertaken. If a young patient, whose only presenting feature is dyspepsia, is going to have a trial of H_2 antagonists anyway, there is little point in performing preceding investigations.

Reminder—if gastric outflow obstruction is suspected, for example the presence of a succussion splash etc., naso-gastric aspiration of stomach contents will be necessary prior to both barium meal and endoscopy.

For suspected gastric malignancy see p. 55.

Small bowel disease

The small bowel may be examined for a wide range of pathologies from malabsorption to malignancy, including inflammatory disease and mechanical problems. The primary investigation is a barium study.

The small bowel meal and the small bowel enema (see glossary of investigations) each have their advocates in different radiology departments. Neither technique has a clear superiority over the other and you will probably get what is offered in your radiology department. If in doubt confer with your radiologists.

Note—*not* 'barium meal and follow through' examination! See list of requests to be avoided at the end of this chapter.

CT can be a useful adjunct examination in the diagnosis of small bowel disease (e.g. Crohn's, where peri-enteric fat proliferation or abscess formation is well shown by CT and will be missed on small bowel contrast examinations). CT is able to demonstrate the relationship of bowel loops and also to examine the mesentery and demonstrate mural thickening. CT may be useful in cases of known small bowel obstruction as it is likely to demonstrate level and cause.

Isotope imaging using the patient's labelled leukocytes (see p. 138) now has a proven role in assessing activity in inflammatory bowel disease (especially Crohn's disease). This is particularly useful when barium studies are equivocal. Similarly, labelled RBCs can be used to detect small bowel bleeding sites, and scintigraphy using pertechnetate has a role in the detection of ectopic gastric mucosa in symptomatic Meckel's diverticula (see p. 139).

Arteriography. Seldom used in the investigation of the small bowel, it may be useful as part of the investigation of occult gastrointestinal blood loss, for example Meckel's diverticulum.

Ultrasound. This can be a useful adjunct (but only an adjunct) in the detection of complications of small bowel disease such as fluid collections and inflammatory bowel masses. It can aid management by discriminating between these two entities. Ultrasound can demonstrate abnormal mural thickening and it has been proposed that it be used for this purpose in the surveillance of chronic inflammatory small bowel disease, to decide which patients require further investigation. This is a little controversial and has not been widely implemented.

Colonic disease

The colon can be examined either by barium enema or colonoscopy. Of the two, colonoscopy has a considerably higher mortality and morbidity rate but has the advantage that detected lesions can be biopsied. Both can be extremely demanding examinations particularly in old, frail, and incontinent patients. Risks in barium enema relate chiefly to perforation, particularly if recent biopsy has been performed. Barium enema therefore, is not performed within seven days of a deep (sigmoidoscopic) biopsy. Superficial biopsy from a colonoscope or flexible sigmoidoscope is less hazardous.

Despite these rather negative comments both examinations are diagnostically effective. Following adequate bowel preparation a double contrast barium enema gives a good overview of the large bowel and is capable of excluding small mucosal lesions. The severity and extent of mucosal changes, for example inflammatory colitis, tend to be underestimated by barium enema as compared to colonoscopy.

Diverticular disease

This is a very common disease in the western world and '? diverticulosis/diverticulitis' is a common reason for requesting a barium enema. As the disease is so common, particularly in the elderly population, simply making the diagnosis of diverticular disease alone is hardly worthwhile, a trial of therapy would suffice. However, frequently the unstated request is to exclude accompanying, more sinister pathology. As change in bowel habit would be a symptom common to diverticular disease or carcinoma this is very reasonable. Barium enema is the examination of choice, probably in combination with flexible sigmoidoscopy. Great distortion of the lower colon can be produced by diverticular disease and the two examinations are often complementary. It is worth noting that it can be extremely difficult to exclude a polyp or carcinoma in a segment of bowel severely involved by diverticular disease.

Subacute and chronic colitis

Active disease. The patient will usually require some preparation to ensure a clean bowel. The radiologist will need to know how severe the patient's current symptoms are when deciding on this. A double contrast enema (p. 31) will usually be performed. It may be possible to differentiate between ulcerative colitis and Crohn's disease, but in a significant number of cases, it will be impossible to decide on radiological grounds alone. Patients will usually undergo flexible sigmoidoscopy (or colonoscopy) and biopsy in addition to the enema.

Longstanding colitis, ? malignancy. In this case, the patient needs a high quality double contrast barium enema with full preparation. Alternatively these patients can be managed with regular colonoscopy and biopsy to detect early malignant change. In fact, recent evidence indicates that surveillance by either method is largely a waste of time and the reward is unlikely to justify the effort.

Gut malignancy

The primary investigation for malignancy of the upper GIT or colon is either direct inspection via endoscopy, or double contrast barium examination. Clinical presentation should suggest the appropriate area for investigation.

Ultrasound departments are frequently asked to scan patients '? GIT malignancy'. Although ultrasound may demonstrate bowel malignancy by showing abnormal masses with thickened bowel walls and an irregular, abnormal lumen within, it is not the primary investigation. Once bowel malignancy has been diagnosed by other means it is quite reasonable to use ultrasound to check for liver metastases.

Chronic/intermittent GIT bleeding

If bleeding from the GIT is proven, investigation should be targeted, if possible, to that end of the GIT most likely to yield results: for example upper GIT for melaena, colon for bright red rectal bleeding. The upper GIT is examined by endoscopy or barium meal and the colon by barium enema or colonoscopy.

If a patient is bleeding actively but not catastrophically, an investigation sequence can be employed as outlined in the emergency imaging section for acute GI bleeding, for example arteriography and/or scintigraphy.

Suspected gallstones

See under 'acute cholecystitis' (above). Similar comments apply to patients with dyspepsia/RUQ pain where gallstones are suspected. Ultrasound is the method of choice and oral chole-cystography will seldom, if ever, be indicated.

Chronic pancreatitis

Ultrasound is the primary investigation method and easily demonstrates the gross changes of diffuse disease, but early morphological changes may be subtle and, if the disease is focal, may be difficult to distinguish from malignancy. Endoscopic ultrasound (using an ultrasound transducer mounted on the distal end of a special endoscope) is not yet widely available, but gives good detail of pancreatic parenchyma through the adjacent stomach wall.

ERCP. Endoscopic cannulation of the pancreatic duct and subsequent contrast injection defines the morphology of the pancreatic duct system. This is a sensitive method of diagnosing early changes of chronic pancreatitis.

CT gives little advantage over ultrasound and ERCP in combination, but may better show extrapancreatic disease and is appropriate for patients not adequately imaged by ultrasound.

Pancreatic malignancy

Ultrasound is the primary investigation method. Better definition of the pancreatic mass may be obtained by CT or MRI and certain features such as extension around the superior mesenteric vessels (a sign of malignancy) will be better appreciated on CT, as will involvement of splenic or portal veins.

Frequently pancreatic mass lesions have non-specific appearances on cross-sectional imaging and require biopsy.

ERCP is used to show duct involvement by pancreatic masses, particularly pancreatic head neoplasms which commonly involve both pancreatic and common bile ducts.

Arteriography, arterioportography (the portal venous phase of a mesenteric angiogram) and, more recently, colour flow doppler, are used to delineate adjacent major vessels in an attempt to assess resectability. However, tumours can only be classed as non-resectable on imaging grounds when there is obvious invasion of adjacent tissues or vessels.

Endocrine tumours

These can be extremely difficult to diagnose because they are frequently multiple and small. It is suggested that you discuss an investigation plan with your own radiologists as this is likely to involve ultrasound, contrast-enhanced CT, possibly arteriography with or without venous sampling and, most accurate of all, intraoperative ultrasound imaging. MRI, where available, may be useful.

Diffuse parenchymal liver disease

This is usually suggested by physical examination and the presence of abnormal LFTs. Ultrasound and CT may confirm diffuse liver disease and give some clue to aetiology, for example irregularity of outline and caudate lobe hypertrophy in cirrhosis. Additional information concerning portal hypertension may also be obtained, for example demonstration of varices and abnormal portal venous flow on colour-flow Doppler. Very few findings in the imaging of generalized liver disease are so specific that biopsy is not performed. Diffuse disorders of the biliary tree, for example sclerosing cholangitis, require contrast cholangiography (usually ERCP).

Focal liver abnormality

In practice this frequently means ? liver metastases. Ultrasound is the primary investigation method for liver metastases, but small lesions may be missed, particularly if the patient is not a good subject for ultrasound examination. Your radiologist will probably advise you if further investigation—usually CT—is indicated. There are now sophisticated CT techniques involving intravenous and even intra-arterial contrast which may be used specifically in the hunt for metastases from particular known primaries. Your radiologist will select the most appropriate CT examination, providing he/she has the necessary clinical information from you. If you are going to investigate by CT anyway, there is no need to perform ultrasound as well. Remember that both ultrasound and CT show morphological changes; a definitive diagnosis requires biopsy.

MRI is effective in demonstrating focal liver lesions and in some, for example haemangioma, specific appearances will occur on appropriate echo sequences. MRI is not yet widely enough available in this country to be used for the primary diagnosis of focal liver abnormalities such as hepatic metastases. It is usually reserved for problem solving when a focal liver abnormality has been demonstrated by some other technique, providing a non-invasive alternative to biopsy.

Solitary liver lesions can cause diagnostic problems. They may have characteristic appearances on ultrasound, CT, MRI, or nuclear medicine, but frequently appearances do not permit confident diagnosis and biopsy is required. As mentioned above, haemangioma is an exception and this can often be confidently diagnosed with specific contrast-enhanced CT techniques, MRI and scintigraphy.

Requests to be avoided

1. 'Dysphagia—gastrografin swallow'. As mentioned above this is dangerous, as inhalation of this hyperosmolar medium can cause pulmonary problems, particularly pulmonary oedema. Similarly, high density barium (the kind used in routine barium meal examinations) will cause problems as its particle size prevents adequate clearing from the lungs by expectoration. Aspiration can cause acute respiratory distress and even chronic fibrosis. Low osmolar water-soluble contrast is the medium of choice and hopefully this is what will be used in your radiology department, whatever the request card says.

2. '? Small bowel pathology—barium meal and follow through please'. This is now an obsolete examination. A satisfactory

small bowel examination cannot be combined with the routine double contrast barium meal. Examination of the small bowel requires specialized techniques (see glossary of investigations).

3. '? Bowel Ca—ultrasound please'. As mentioned above this is inappropriate as a first-line investigation. Ultrasound of the liver looking for metastases is appropriate for patients in whom bowel malignancy has been diagnosed by endoscopy or double contrast barium examination.

4. '? Gallstones—ultrasound negative—oral cholecystogram please'. As mentioned above there is no justification for this request.

In patients with a normal ultrasound in whom there remains a strong clinical suspicion of gallbladder disease, a HIDA scan is performed. This may show delayed or absent filling of the gall-bladder due to chronic cholecystitis or the relatively rare acute condition of acalculous cholecystitis.

5. 'Admitted today with ? Acute pancreatitis—ultrasound please'. As discussed above this is inappropriate. The diagnosis of pancreatitis is made on clinical and biochemical grounds. Imaging techniques are reserved for the complications of the disease, and better results are obtained after a short delay.

7

Genito-urinary tract

The investigation of urological problems is one of those clinical areas long bedevilled by established medical culture and historical precedence. But times have changed. The era when the IVU was the only investigation method available is over, although some clinicians still place inappropriate emphasis on this examination.

We start the chapter with an outline of the main investigations used, listing pros and cons. These are generalizations.

1. Plain abdominal radiography may show calculi. Likely to show a plethora of other calcifications not in urinary tract.

2. IVU. Shows if calcification detected on the plain film is within renal tract. Allows you to count number of functioning kidneys (0, 1 or 2), but not to estimate absolute renal function or split function. Does show the urothelium in detail (which ultrasound, CT, and isotopes do not). Misses lots of small renal masses. Does not differentiate cystic from solid renal masses Approximately 1 in 40 000 patients will have life threatening contrast medium reactions, and many more will suffer minor reactions. The bowel preparation can also be unpleasant for some patients.

3. Ultrasound. Good for detecting mass lesions. Differentiates solid from cystic but does not distinguish between the various solid pathologies. Demonstrates calculi, but tiny ones can be missed. Does not accurately delineate peri-renal fascial planes. Bad for the demonstration of urothelial lesions. Good for demonstrating dilated collecting systems, but dilatation does not necessarily imply obstruction.

4. CT. Good for demonstrating mass lesions and relationships to capsule and fascial planes, etc. Some mass lesions may have specific features on CT, for example fat content of angiomyolipoma. Poor sensitivity for small urothelial lesions.

5. Isotopes. Excellent for function, especially the detection of obstruction. Nuclear medicine techniques are of limited use when renal function is very poor (see below under renal failure). Poor spatial resolution for mass lesions. DMSA good for differentiating normal tissue (especially big columns of Bertin) from tumour. Of no use for urothelial lesions. DMSA is the method of choice for detecting renal scarring (see p. 137).

6. Arteriography. Ideal for demonstrating the anatomy of renal vascular disease (with isotopes for function). Good at showing pathological circulation, but this is very non-specific, i.e. inflammation (e.g. xanthogranulomatous pyelonephritis) and tumour can be indistinguishable.

Having read the above you will see that no single investigation is likely to provide enough information for anything but straightforward problems. Pinpoint the problem, define the questions and choose the investigations appropriately.

Emergency imaging

Renal/ureteric colic

Imaging is often used to decide whether or not to admit the patient. Even if the patient needs to be admitted for symptomatic relief you will want to confirm that the symptoms originate in the renal tract.

The plain AXR is performed in the first instance. This may show the presence of calculi but will not prove that they lie within the renal tract. Almost invariably an IVU will be necessary to obtain this proof and may demonstrate delayed drainage or acute obstruction.

In most centres an acute, limited IVU will be performed. A single full length, post micturition film taken 20 minutes after the injection of contrast medium is likely to provide all the information necessary in this acute phase. A normal limited IVU in a patient who is still in pain effectively excludes renal colic as the cause.

Should the acute IVU reveal a poorly functioning kidney, further investigation is necessary. Delayed films may be taken, or an ultrasound scan performed if there is inadequate opacification of the collecting system. If obstruction is not demonstrated then consider other causes of renal pain such as pyelonephritis, renal vein thrombosis, or arterial infarction, which can present in the same manner.

Ultrasound is also useful in excluding disease in neighbouring organs. For example, in patients presenting with right upper quadrant pain it may be difficult to differentiate between pain of gallbladder and renal origin, despite what the surgical texts may say. As the gallbladder often lies immediately anterior to the right kidney this is not surprising.

Acute obstruction

This follows on from the section above, as acute obstruction may be present in patients with ureteric colic. The IVU is the primary investigation and, if the opacification is inadequate, or bilateral obstruction is suspected (see acute renal failure below), ultrasound is performed. In addition to IVU and ultrasound, isotope renography will confirm the presence and degree of renal obstruction, and quantify relative renal function.

Having confirmed obstruction you will want to know the level; this will often be shown on the IVU and less frequently on ultrasound. If a kidney is shown to be obstructed but the level and nature of the obstruction is still undetermined, antegrade or retrograde pyelography may be necessary (see glossary of investigations).

Renal trauma

See section on non-skeletal trauma, Chapter 13.

Acute renal failure

The diagnosis of acute renal failure will have been made on the basis of anuria or oliguria and deteriorating biochemical indices of renal function. Investigation is aimed at demonstrating cause. Ultrasound is the first investigation method, primarily to exclude bilateral renal obstruction or bladder outflow obstruction. Pathology such as unsuspected adult polycystic disease may occasionally be discovered in this way. Other ultrasound changes in acute renal failure tend to be non-specific.

Colour-flow and quantitative Doppler studies may be useful in excluding vascular compromise although many patients with renovascular disease have bilateral problems making interpretation of the Doppler indices difficult.

In patients with acute renal failure an IVU can be hazardous, and, if renal failure is advanced, is unlikely to be informative due to poor visualization of the renal tract.

Cases of vascular compromise may need angiography or venography after other causes for renal failure have been excluded. You will need to consult your radiologist.

Nuclear medicine in established renal failure. Renal scintigraphy seldom adds useful information, but a short dynamic study will at least confirm that the kidneys are perfused. It is important to note that renography should not be used to *exclude* obstruction as a cause of renal failure. Stick to ultrasound for this purpose (the collecting systems should be dilated in obstruction sufficiently severe and longstanding to cause renal failure).

Deteriorating function in a transplant kidney

A failing transplant kidney can be managed using the investigation plan as above. Ultrasound is used to demonstrate the presence or absence of dilatation of the collecting system and isotopes may be used to calculate indices of vascularization and exclude obstruction. As the two most common problems encountered are rejection and immunosuppressant toxicity, renal biopsy is the single most useful investigation. Your radiologist may offer ultrasound guidance for accurate biopsy with reduction of the complication rate.

Isotope studies are widely used to monitor function in transplanted kidneys, but most of the indices quoted are non-specific and often unable to differentiate between, for example, acute tubular necrosis and rejection. Even when serial studies are available, it will usually be necessary to resort to biopsy (or a trial of therapy).

Acute pyelonephritis

The diagnosis will usually be made on clinical presentation and examination of an MSU. A KUB (p. 153) may be useful to demonstrate the presence of associated calculi and, if stones are present, it would be reasonable to proceed to ultrasound to make sure that there is no upper tract obstruction. In patients who fail to settle on the appropriate antibiotic therapy, ultrasound is useful in excluding the presence of renal or perinephric abscess. The IVU is of little use in the acute phase but once the patient's symptoms have settled, may be used to show the scarring and calyceal distortion of chronic pyelonephritis (see below).

'Cold' imaging'

Haematuria

Bleeding in the urinary tract must, by definition, involve the urothelium. Therefore an IVU is the first line of investigation, often combined with cystoscopy. The IVU should be performed first as, if there is any suspicion of an ureteric lesion, retrograde pyelography can be performed at the time of cystoscopy. Ultrasound is useful in delineating renal masses, including some which are invisible on IVU. In some centres, ultrasound is assuming a more important role in the investigation of haematuria, and certainly it is capable of detecting quite small bladder tumours. It is important to remember that even a good quality

IVU can miss bladder pathology—hence the importance of cystoscopy.

Prostatism

The real questions are whether there is bladder outflow obstruction, and whether the upper tracts are dilated.

Both these questions can be satisfactorily answered by ultrasound. Bladder size, wall thickness, and prostatic bulk can be assessed by transabdominal scanning. Following micturition the residual volume can be estimated. Upper tract dilatation is clearly demonstrated by ultrasound, and by inference we conclude that it is secondary to outflow obstruction. There is no justification for an IVU in simple prostatism. Estimation of voiding rate, accurate residual volume, and bladder pressures can be obtained at voiding cystometrography. Abnormalities of detrusor or sphincter function are more complex and are usually investigated in specialist units.

Prostatic neoplasm

Investigation will depend upon surgical practice in your hospital, many surgeons performing their own biopsies. The only useful imaging is transrectal ultrasound (plus biopsy). In proven cases of carcinoma, a case can be made for bone scanning as part of the staging process, and a scan is certainly indicated in any patient with bone pain.

Incontinence

Imaging has little to offer. Stress incontinence used to be investigated by the stress cystogram. This examination involved bladder opacification with contrast instilled via a catheter and lateral images obtained of the bladder at rest, straining, and during micturition. The object was to demonstrate abnormal changes in the angle between bladder floor and proximal urethra.

Results correlate poorly with symptoms and this technique is seldom used now.

Renal mass

Ultrasound is the first line of investigation. It will differentiate between simple cysts and solid tumours, and in cases of doubt, CT will be helpful. Angiography is seldom indicated, and can lead to confusion, chronic inflammatory lesions mimicking tumours on occasions.

Percutaneous biopsy can be performed under ultrasound or CT guidance. This must be performed with care as renal masses can be highly vascular. The need for biopsy is questionable; most tumours are confidently diagnosed on ultrasound or CT.

Once a renal carcinoma has been diagnosed secondary investigation will be directed at answering the following questions:

1. Is the tumour resectable?
2. Is the other kidney functioning normally?
3. Is there any evidence of distant spread?

In general, imaging correlates poorly with the surgeon's ability to resect the tumour. Spread through fascial planes or invasion of the renal veins or IVC may affect surgical management. The presence of a tumour in the venous system can usually be demonstrated by ultrasound but perinephric tissue planes are best seen on CT.

Synchronous tumours in the other kidney can be excluded with a good level of accuracy by either ultrasound or CT, and function of the contra-lateral kidney is best judged by scintigraphy. So, an IVU is of little use unless there is any question that the tumour is of urothelial origin and not a renal cell carcinoma.

The presence of lung metastases is the one finding that usually militates against surgery (unless intervention is necessary for other reasons, e.g. persisting gross haematuria). The presence of early lung metastases is undoubtedly best shown by CT, preceded by chest X-ray to exclude obvious larger metastases.

Patients with persisting significant haematuria who are considered inoperable because of local invasion or distant metastases can be treated by arterial embolization. This will have to be discussed with your radiologists.

Chronic renovascular disease

This usually presents clinically as hypertension, (especially when refractory to treatment or occurring in younger patients) or as declining renal function (see acute renal failure above). Reduced renal function following ACE-inhibitor therapy may suggest the diagnosis. It has to be said that there is no single easy test. Ultrasound is commonly used as an initial screening procedure to demonstrate small kidneys or a discrepancy in renal sizes. Doppler studies may be useful but are difficult to interpret and are not universally reliable. Isotope renography is a useful screening test, but the changes seen in renovascular disease are non-specific.

Angiography remains the gold standard and maybe augmented by renal vein renin assays. Angiography is obviously a necessary precursor to angioplasty. (See glossary, p. 145.)

Polycystic disease (PCK)

Ultrasound is the first line imaging procedure and often all that is necessary. In adolescence and early adulthood the results of a negative or intermediate scan (i.e. one or two cysts demonstrable) need to be viewed with a little caution. There is no difficulty in making the positive diagnosis when multiple cysts of varying size are seen in both kidneys (and possibly in the liver and pancreas too). Two common complications of adult PCK disease are bleeding and infection. Both can be extremely difficult to localize. Ultrasound or CT may demonstrate abnormal cyst contents which can be aspirated with imaging guidance. Isotope scanning using labelled RBCs or WBCs may locate the problem area.

Chronic pyelonephritis

An IVU will show scarring and the underlying deformity of the renal calyces. Similar information can be obtained from careful ultrasound scanning, although the spatial resolution is not as good. DMSA scanning is probably the best method for demonstrating scarring, and gives an estimate of relative renal function. For a fuller discussion of reflux nephropathy and the role of other imaging techniques, see the section on paediatric UTI (p. 129).

Urethral disease

All urethral disease, for example ? trauma, ? stricture, ? diverticulum tend to be investigated by ascending and descending urethrography although in some centres surgeons perform urethroscopy as a first line investigation. Recently there has been some interest in urethrosonography, an ultrasound technique in which the urethra is distended with fluid. This is not widely available, although it is claimed to give better information about peri-urethral tissues. Ultrasound is the only investigation in Peyronie's disease that has been shown to be of any use, although the clinical impact of any imaging in this condition seems limited.

Vasculogenic impotence

There is a great diversity in opinion concerning the appropriate investigations for vasculogenic impotence at the present time. The techniques include arteriography, cavernosography with or without papaverine stimulation and manometry. A complex subject developing rapidly. Consult your radiologist!!

Scrotal disease

Investigation of scrotal disease is very simple to outline. Patients you suspect of having malignancy or unresponsive inflammatory disease need scrotal ultrasound. Remember that not all testicular tumours present as painless masses and that some early tumours may not be palpable despite causing symptoms.

In adult patients that are suspected of torsion, ultrasound imaging is of no use as the appearances are very similar to those of acute epididymitis. Colour-flow Doppler and spectral analysis may help, and certainly normal flow effectively excludes infarction, but the best investigation method for torsion is an isotope perfusion scan. However, probably the most appropriate line of action is no investigation at all. If you think that your patient has suffered torsion of the testis, intervention not investigation, is required.

8

Obstetrics, gynaecology, and breast

It is difficult to imagine any area of medicine where a single imaging technique has had such an impact on everyday practice as has ultrasound in obstetrics and gynaecology. Techniques using ionizing radiation are seldom required, and in this chapter it can be assumed that ultrasound is the first choice of investigation, unless otherwise stated.

In transabdominal scanning, a full bladder is essential to give an acoustic 'window' on to the pelvic viscera. However, vaginal probes are now available which provide high resolution images of the uterus and adnexal regions with no preparation.

GYNAECOLOGY

Emergency imaging

Bleeding in early pregnancy

There are two questions to answer. First, is the patient pregnant and second, is the fetus viable?

The gestation sac becomes visible at four to five weeks, but a fetal pole may not be seen until six weeks, and a heartbeat is not reliably detectable until seven weeks (see Table 8.1).

Table 8.1   Ultrasonic landmarks in pregnancy

4–5 weeks	Gestation sac seen
6 weeks	Fetal pole visible
7 weeks	Fetal heart motion seen
8–12 weeks	Crown-rump length used for dating
12 weeks plus	Biparietal diameter used
16–18 weeks	Screening for fetal abnormality
32 weeks plus	Late scans for IUGR or placenta praevia

Therefore, if the initial scan shows a small sac with no visible contents, it will often be impossible to give an opinion concerning viability until a repeat scan shows either no change or a reduction in size of the sac (non-viable), or the appearance of a fetal pole (viable).

Suspected ectopic pregnancy

The only 100 per cent reliable indication of an ectopic gestation is the demonstration of a typical gestation sac and fetus lying outside the uterus; in practice, this is rarely seen.

Most of the signs of an ectopic pregnancy are non-specific, but when seen in a patient with a convincing history, the diagnosis cannot be excluded.

The most useful scan in this clinical context is the one which reveals an intrauterine pregnancy. This almost (but not quite) excludes the possibility of a coexisting ectopic gestation.

'Cold' imaging

Pelvic tumours

Ultrasound will confirm the presence of a mass, and may often indicate its nature. However, CT/MRI will usually be indicated in the diagnosis and staging of pelvic tumours. Don't forget that pelvic masses are not always gynaecological.

Dysfunctional uterine bleeding

Although fibroids can have a characteristic appearance, it is frequently impossible to differentiate between benign and malignant uterine tumours. Cytology or histology remains the definitive diagnostic tool.

Infertility

Ultrasound will allow you to check that the pelvic organs are present and grossly normal and it will sometimes reveal pathology such as endometriosis. Laparoscopic insufflation of coloured dye or, alternatively, hysterosalpingography (p. 138) are necessary to demonstrate tubal patency, although a few enthusiasts use water insufflation with ultrasound monitoring.

Ultrasound also has a role in monitoring follicle development and harvesting of eggs for *in vitro* fertilization. Vaginal probes have proved particularly useful in this respect.

The lost coil

A common problem. Radiography has no place in the initial investigation—the patient needs an ultrasound scan. Apart from the risk of irradiating an early pregnancy, an X-ray will not tell you if a coil seen in the pelvis is within the uterus, embedded in its wall or lying free in the abdominal cavity. Only if the scan fails to reveal the IUCD will it be reasonable to perform radiography to ensure that it is genuinely lost, and has not migrated through the uterine wall (where it may be invisible to ultrasound, lying between loops of bowel).

OBSTETRICS

Emergency imaging

There are lots of obstetric emergencies, but few of them call for urgent imaging. Where it is required, for example to localize the placenta in *ante partum* haemorrhage, ultrasound will be the answer.

'Cold' imaging

Assessment of pelvic adequacy

Pelvimetry is just about the only radiographic technique still used for specifically obstetric purposes, and even this is becoming a relative rarity. Usually requested either during pregnancy when problems are anticipated (e.g. persistent breech) or after a difficult delivery in a patient who intends to have more children. A single lateral view is obtained, with a metal ruler between the patient's legs to allow measurement of the obstetric conjugates from the film.

Ultrasound

The benefits of ultrasound in pregnancy are now accepted, and routine obstetric scanning is practised almost universally. Its advantages are briefly listed here.

1. Gestational age. Ultrasonic measurement of the fetus has been shown to be superior to other methods of predicting the date of delivery. Table 8.1 sets out the parameters used at different stages of pregnancy. Remember that the range of normal becomes broader with increasing gestational age, and this is one of the reasons for performing the first routine scan at 16–18 weeks.

2. Fetal abnormality. Neural tube defects are the most frequently diagnosed anomalies, and scans of the spine performed before 16 weeks have an unacceptably high false negative rate—another reason for routine scanning at 16–18 weeks. Urinary tract abnormalities such as hydronephrosis and gastrointestinal problems are also regularly picked up.

3. Placental site. A low placenta on the early scan is a frequent finding. A second scan at 32 weeks or more will usually confirm

that the placenta has 'migrated' away from the os as the lower segment of the uterus develops. In cases where a true placenta praevia persists, obstetric arrangements can be made accordingly.

4. Fetal growth. Recognition of intrauterine growth retardation requires at least one late scan. Growth of the head tends to be preserved, and so abdominal circumference or the ratio of abdominal and head size are used. A single estimation of abdominal circumference will detect up to 80 per cent of growth-retarded babies.

BREAST DISEASE

This is a short section, not because breast disease is unimportant, but because there are only one or two different presentations requiring imaging.

Two methods are available for imaging the breast—mammography and ultrasound. Thermography enjoyed a vogue, but is now rarely used, and transillumination of the breast using a high intensity light source has only been taken-up in a few centres.

Emergency imaging

There are no true emergencies in breast disease, although any significant breast symptom requires prompt attention.

'Cold' imaging

Breast lump

The decision as to which lumps are significant must clearly rest with the clinician, but when any suspicion is aroused, mammography is the examination of choice. Ultrasound is useful to determine whether a mass is solid or cystic, and to guide drainage or needle biopsy. It is also useful in young, dense breasts, where it may be difficult to demonstrate small lesions using mammography alone.

Remember that mammography has a false negative rate of at least 5 per cent. If a mass is clinically suspicious, a normal mammogram should not stand in the way of excision or needle biopsy. Conversely, a suspicious lesion on mammography requires attention, even when no abnormality is palpable.

Blood-stained nipple discharge

This symptom is more frequently due to duct papilloma than to carcinoma. Mammography will be indicated, and some surgeons will request galactography (p. 138) to confirm the diagnosis.

Breast pain

Cyclical breast discomfort is common, and of itself will seldom be an indication for imaging. However, pain can be the sole presenting symptom of cancer, and when there is any suspicion of tumour, mammography will be the investigation of choice.

Mastitis/breast abscess

When a patient presents with acute pain and inflammation in the breast, the diagnosis of mastitis will normally be a clinical one, at least initially. Mammography requires compression of the breast: the presence of acute inflammation makes this difficult to achieve, and the patient will not thank you for trying. However, ultrasound is a reliable method for detecting the presence of a collection of pus requiring drainage. Abscesses are traditionally drained surgically, but some centres are now using ultrasound-guided aspiration in conjunction with systemic antibiotics with good results.

Remember that carcinoma can occasionally present as acute inflammation, and mammography is indicated when a presumed infective process fails to respond to treatment.

Screening for breast cancer

Whole books can and will be written on this topic. Suffice it to say that large studies in the USA and Scandinavia have suggested a reduction in mortality from breast cancer of up to 40 per cent in populations subjected to regular screening, and given the current rate of around 15 000 deaths per year in the UK from this disease, the attractions of screening are obvious.

The theory is that, since mammography can detect impalpable tumours, routine examination in asymptomatic women should result in earlier diagnosis and hence a better chance of cure. The UK screening programme has initially been limited to women between the ages of 50 and 65, and will be repeated every three years. This may not be the optimal interval, and it remains to be seen if the results will be as good as those in the studies quoted above. Investigations are also under way to determine if there is any benefit to women under the age of 50.

You will come across some patients who require screening, even though they are not in the age group covered by the national programme. These will include women with a personal history of breast cancer, and those with a strong family history of the disease. Mammography is indicated for these patients, although there is some debate over the optimum frequency of screening, and the age at which it should start. There is continuing debate concerning the need for screening in women who are on hormone replacement therapy.

Screening is not without its problems, as we hinted in Chapter 1, and we can expect to see some fairly rigorous cost/benefit analysis of the initial results of the screening programme.

<h1 style="text-align:center">9</h1>

Musculoskeletal system (excluding trauma)

Trauma is considered separately in Chapter 13. In the present chapter we look first at imaging by clinical presentation, and then at the role of radiology in specific diseases. If the selection of topics appears arbitrary, it is because we have chosen those areas which most frequently generate imaging requests, appropriate or otherwise. Musculoskeletal problems in children are covered in Chapter 14.

Imaging by clinical presentation

Neck pain

For the otherwise fit middle-aged to elderly patient with a painful neck, radiography has little to offer. The changes of cervical spondylosis are seen just as often in asymptomatic as in symptomatic patients over the age of 60, and it is very rare for the X-ray to reveal a more sinister cause for the pain. If there are signs or symptoms of nerve root compression, oblique films may show narrowing of the exit foramina by osteophytes, but this is only relevant if surgical relief is contemplated, and in this case the patient needs cervical radiculography or CT/MRI scanning, whatever the plain films look like. There is certainly no point asking for repeat films every time a patient suffers an exacerbation of their symptoms.

Naturally, if there is good reason to suspect serious pathology such as metastasis or infection, then plain films are justified.

Frozen shoulder/capsulitis/supraspinatus tendonitis

Frozen shoulder often develops for no apparent reason, persists for a considerable number of months and then gets better. Plain radiography will inevitably be performed, but has little effect on the course of events, other than excluding more sinister causes for the pain. The diagnosis will be made clinically, and the shoulder is usually radiographically normal, or shows non-specific degenerative change. An exception is the calcification seen adjacent to the greater tuberosity in the chronic/healing stage of rotator cuff lesions.

Arthrography, either conventional or combined with CT, gives a very nice demonstration of rotator cuff tears, as can ultrasound in experienced hands. All of these techniques will probably be replaced by MRI, where it is available. It is only worthwhile requesting any of these investigations if your orthopaedic surgeon feels that the result will influence treatment.

Low back pain

Plain radiography of the lumbar spine probably causes more unnecessary irradiation of gonads and bone marrow than any other single request. The chief justification for radiography is to exclude serious pathology such as tumour or infection. In most cases, especially in young patients, this possibility will only arise if there are specific additional symptoms or signs, or if the condition fails to respond to conservative treatment.

Most back pain originates in the soft tissues. In acute disc prolapse the plain films will frequently be normal, and by the time changes of a chronic disc lesion are seen, the patient's symptoms may well be originating from another site. Degenerative changes (spondylosis) are a normal feature after the age of 50 or so, and their presence or absence correlates poorly with symptoms, and is of little relevance to management.

Spondylolysis (defect in the pars interarticularis, usually of L4 or L5) and spondylolysthesis (a spondylolysis with forward slip of a vertebra on the one below) are relatively common radiological findings. The defects may be visible on routine lumbar spine views, but oblique projections are frequently required. These involve extra radiation for the patient, and should not be requested routinely in the investigation of back pain. The fact that a patient has a pars defect does not mean that it is the source of the pain. Scintigraphy can be useful here—increased uptake at the site of a defect suggests that it is indeed responsible, and this will help in the selection of patients for operative treatment.

Low back pain with symptoms or signs of root involvement

The majority of patients coming to surgery for their low back pain do so because of symptoms and signs of nerve root irritation or compression. They will invariably have had plain films taken already, and there is nothing to be gained from repeating them. When symptoms are severe enough to require surgical relief (and only then), the patient needs a 'proper' investigation —in this case a lumbar radiculogram (see p. 141) or, increasingly, a CT or MRI scan.

Acute cord compression presenting with long tract signs (or saddle anaesthesia and loss of bladder control in the case of the cauda equina), is a genuine radiological emergency. Do not delay orthopaedic or neurosurgical referral in order to obtain plain films—the patient will need radiculography or myelography (see pp. 140–1, also Chapter 10), although CT/MRI will probably be the first choice where it is available. Plain films may be required, but they can be performed at the same time as the more definitive examination.

Vertebral collapse

A common problem. Questions we are usually asked are 'how recent is the collapse' and 'is it due to osteoporosis or to tumour?' Sadly, the answer often has to be that we don't know —imaging has a very limited role to play. Plain films are indicated, and if they show an obvious destructive lesion in the vertebra, especially in the pedicle, or if there are typical meta-static lesions elsewhere in the vicinity, they may be helpful. Once a vertebral body has collapsed, it can be very difficult to determine the cause—osteoporosis, metastasis, myeloma, and even infection can all result in similar appearances. Some assessment of the age of the lesion may be possible, but this is a subjective judgement.

Scintigraphy is considerably more sensitive than radiography in detecting crush fractures, but it will not identify the underlying aetiology unless it reveals unsuspected lesions elsewhere which have a characteristic scintigraphic or radiographic appearance. It is also less helpful than is sometimes supposed in putting an age to vertebral fractures. If a crush fracture is cold on scanning, then it is safe to say that it is old, almost certainly older than six months. However, if as is normally the case the activity is increased, it does not necessarily mean that the fracture is recent; they can remain hot for eighteen months or more. It is unlikely that any kind of imaging actually has much effect on management in these elderly patients.

Vague joint pains—? arthritis

Plain films will usually be indicated if the pains seem to be joint-related and persistent. Remember though, that in many of the arthritides (see the section on imaging specific conditions below) radiographic changes occur relatively late in the disease process. If there is good cause to suspect a significant arthritis, and if plain films are unhelpful or the symptoms are widespread and you don't know where to start, bone scintigraphy is a good method for demonstrating the presence or absence of disease and identifying those joints which are active. Scintigraphy will also document response to treatment, but we doubt if this is ever of much real use in management.

Painful knee

We report a lot of radiographs on young patients with non-specific knee pain, and they are nearly always normal. As with the lumbar spine, the pain arises in the soft tissues in most of these patients, and the radiographs simply serve to exclude relatively uncommon bony lesions such as tumours or osteo-chondritis diseccans.

Patients with suspected meniscal tears are likely to require arthroscopy, arthrography, or, best of all, an MRI scan. Plain films will not help.

Osgood–Schlatter's disease, see p. 133.

Imaging in specific conditions

The arthritides

Osteoarthritis (OA). Above a certain age, osteoarthritis (OA) can be regarded as normal and may or may not be the cause of the patient's symptoms. We get a lot of requests for plain radiography in elderly patients saying, for example, 'pain in knee—? OA'. Of course, they almost invariably do have OA, and it doesn't alter management one jot. As in the cervical spine, it is exceedingly uncommon to turn up an unexpected cause for the pain. Radiography does help when patients have pain which could be coming either from hip or lumbar spine—a not in-frequent occurrence.

While a single plain film may be justifiable where there is clinical doubt, or where there is reason to suspect other pathology (e.g. in patients with a known primary malignancy), once the diagnosis of OA is made there is no point in repeated examina-tions to monitor progress. When surgery is contemplated, the decision to operate will be made on clinical, not radiological grounds.

Plain radiography is reasonable when there is suspicion of an intra-articular loose body. In this case arthrography may also be required (or CT/MRI) if plain films are inconclusive.

Rheumatoid arthritis. Plain radiography will always be the first imaging investigation when rheumatoid arthritis (RA) is sus-pected, but it must be remembered that in the early stages of the disease the films may be normal or show only minimal change. Initial diagnosis will usually be made on clinical and serological grounds. Radiography comes into its own in following progress and detecting complications.

As mentioned above, if there is doubt about the diagnosis of arthropathy, or its extent, joint scintigraphy is indicated.

When a patient with known RA is to undergo general anaesthesia or endoscopy, radiography of the cervical spine should be requested, including lateral views in flexion/extension, to detect any instability, particularly at the atlanto–axial level.

Ankylosing spondylitis and rheumatoid variants. Most of the comments made in the previous section apply equally here. The radiographic diagnosis of sacroiliitis can be difficult, and CT is indicated when plain films are inconclusive.

Quantitative scintigraphy: it is possible to quantify the uptake of standard bone scanning agents in the SIJs and arrive at a sacro-iliac index. Although the index is raised in active disease, the technique is of limited value in individual patients due to overlap between normal and abnormal ranges.

Gout. In gout it is not unusual for radiographs to be normal— erosions and tophi are only seen in established disease. Initial diagnosis will rest on clinical and biochemical findings.

Malignant disease

Metastatic

If you are screening a patient with a known primary malignancy for metastatic disease then scintigraphy is the method of choice. It will frequently detect metastases long before the radiograph becomes abnormal. This does not mean that all patients with malignant disease should have bone scintigraphy as part of the staging process, even if the tumour is one of those (lung, breast, prostate, kidney, thyroid) which commonly metastasize to bone.

For example, there is now general agreement that scintigraphy is not indicated in early breast cancer, as the pick-up rate is so low. Your radiologists and oncologists will doubtless have protocols for the investigation of different tumours—make sure you know about them so that you can avoid unnecessary tests.

If a patient with malignant disease develops bone pain, scintigraphy is again the investigation of choice. Remember though that radiography of hot spots will often be required to exclude a benign cause for the uptake, a reflection of the lack of specificity of bone scanning.

Myeloma

Myeloma is generally bracketed with metastasis when it comes to radiological diagnosis, as the appearances can be identical. The important difference is that bone scintigraphy can be normal in patients with myeloma; this is unusual in metastatic disease. When imaging is required then the radiographic skeletal survey is probably the first choice: but when *is* imaging required? Diagnosis is founded on plasma electrophoresis and marrow examination. Focal treatment will only be considered for symptomatic lesions, in which case you only need to examine the region that hurts. So *you will seldom need either a scan or skeletal survey.*

Primary bone tumours

Plain radiography will usually suggest the diagnosis of tumour, although it will not always be possible to say exactly what type. Radiologists and pathologists work very closely together in making the final diagnosis. The need for further imaging will depend on the histology and the proposed management. CT scanning is now established as the method of choice for defining the extent of the tumour pre-operatively, as plain films (and scintigraphy) can be misleading. MRI will almost certainly have a major role here, once it is widely available.

Soft tissue tumours

When patients present with a soft tissue mass, excision and/or biopsy will usually be indicated. In those cases where the mass is so obviously innocent (e.g. lipoma) that biopsy is not required, then it is equally unnecessary to request imaging. For some tumours a plain film may be indicated to exclude bony involvement.

As for the mass itself, ultrasound will confirm its presence and give some idea of its extent; it will seldom give much information about its nature, other than differentiating solid from cystic. In the case of large lesions, or those in surgically awkward situations, CT or MRI will be needed. CT and ultrasound will allow guided percutaneous biopsy to be performed.

Bone and joint infection

Osteomyelitis and septic arthritis

In early bone or joint infection plain films are frequently normal. Bone scintigraphy will reveal increased uptake well before radiographic changes set in, but it will not prove that the hot spot is due to infection—material must be obtained for culture. If this is impossible, a labelled leukocyte scan should be requested. In patients thought to have chronic low-grade infection, a gallium scan may well be more useful—discuss this with your radiologist before making the request.

Again, in difficult cases, CT/MRI can be very helpful in confirming the extent of disease and guiding drainage/diagnostic aspiration of pus.

Painful arthroplasty

This is likely to be due to loosening or infection.

Infection. The definitive diagnosis depends on obtaining material from the suspect area, but imaging is usually requested first. Plain films will always be obtained, but are of limited use. Bone scintigraphy should be requested. If it is normal, then there is no indication for further imaging as infection is very unlikely. When activity is increased, the pattern of uptake may help to differentiate between loosening and infection, but often a further scan will be needed using either gallium or labelled leukocytes. Find out what your local policy is.

Loosening. This is usually a diagnosis of exclusion when infection has been ruled out (see previous paragraph).

However, positive evidence may be obtained from arthrography. If there is loosening, contrast medium will be seen between bone and the prosthesis. Fluoroscopic screening of the hip during passive movement may also confirm the presence of loosening.

Metabolic bone disease

Osteoporosis

Although we often find ourselves reporting 'widespread reduction in bone density', the diagnosis of osteoporosis from plain films is very subjective. If you want to know what the bone density is, you have to measure it. There are methods of using CT to do this, but dedicated bone densitometers are now becoming more widely available and, along with hormone replacement, will have an increasing role in prophylaxis.

Hyperparathyroidism/osteomalacia/renal osteodystrophy

Traditionally, radiography has been used in the diagnosis of metabolic bone disease, but bone scintigraphy is more sensitive. It is questionable whether imaging adds very much to biochemical monitoring in the absence of localized skeletal symptoms. Plain films in symptomatic patients may reveal, for example Looser's zones in osteomalacia or brown tumours in patients with hyperparathyroidism.

Paget's disease

Although the plain film changes are often characteristic, it can be impossible to differentiate between Paget's and sclerotic metastases. This problem most frequently arises in elderly men where prostatic carcinoma is either suspected or proven. Scintigraphy is more sensitive than radiography in revealing lesions due to either pathology, but will not always distinguish between them. Biochemistry (acid phosphatase, prostate-specific antigen) often will, although biopsy may still be necessary.

Scintigraphy is the method of choice for revealing the extent of active disease in a patient known to have Paget's disease, should this be thought clinically relevant.

10

Head and neck (including central nervous system)

Because this chapter deals with an anatomical region rather than a body system, the list of contents lacks a common theme, and may look somewhat arbitrary. Although we have included the CNS, neuroradiology is a specialty in its own right, and coverage is necessarily limited to the bare essentials. This chapter contains advice on imaging strategy in commonly occurring conditions, although you will usually wish to discuss acute neurological/neurosurgical cases with the radiologist before requesting any but the most basic imaging procedures. Three general points are worth making before dealing with specific clinical problems.

1. Undue reliance is often placed on the skull X-ray as an indicator of intracranial pathology. Remember that a normal plain film excludes nothing, and even when it is abnormal, the changes seen are likely to be non-specific. In other words, when there is clinical suspicion of intracranial disease, the patient will require the definitive examination (CT or MRI scan) whatever the plain films show.

2. Requests for isotope brain scanning have been much reduced by the arrival of CT with its greater sensitivity and ability to demonstrate detailed intracranial anatomy. Standard scintigraphy will seldom, if ever, be the procedure of choice when you are looking for focal cerebral pathology. However, new radiopharmaceuticals allow us to map the distribution of cerebral blood flow, and scintigraphy may well find a new role in neuroimaging in the fairly near future.

3. When we recommend CT scanning, MRI will frequently be equally applicable. Where both modalities are available, the radiologist will usually decide which is the more appropriate.

Emergency imaging

Head injury

See Chapter 13, p. 111.

Cerebrovascular accident (stroke)

CT is the first choice investigation, usually allowing you to differentiate between haemorrhage and infarction, a distinction which is frequently difficult to make clinically. CT will also occasionally reveal unsuspected pathology such as a tumour. The role of angiography in stroke is contentious, and is outside the scope of this book.

Subarachnoid haemorrhage

CT is the first investigation to confirm the presence of blood in the subarachnoid space, and may indicate the site of origin. Angiography is required to delineate the anatomy prior to surgery.

Meningitis

The initial diagnosis is based on clinical findings and CSF analysis. When you suspect complications such as abscess, subdural collection or hydrocephalus, CT will be indicated.

Acute spinal cord compression

After plain films, MRI will be the examination of choice. Where MRI is not available, myelography is indicated.

Sudden loss of vision

Most ocular causes of visual loss will be diagnosed on ophthal-mological examination. In circumstances where direct fundo-scopy is not possible, CT and ultrasound are both capable of demonstrating intraocular pathology such as retinal detachment, haemorrhage, and tumour. Where the problem is thought to be behind the retina, involving optic nerves, optic radiations or occipital cortex, CT is the examination of choice, although in most circumstances MRI will be equally applicable.

? Penetrating eye injury

See visceral trauma, p. 117.

Acute upper airway obstruction

The patient will usually be a child. See p. 122.

'Cold' imaging

Suspected cerebral space occupying lesion

Don't forget the CXR in any patient suspected of harbouring a cerebral tumour. It may reveal a source of cerebral metastases, or an infective source for an abscess. Otherwise, CT is the first and often the only imaging investigation needed. Plain films are of limited value, as is scintigraphy (see above). In some cases, angiography will still be indicated, especially when surgery is being considered, and the radiologist may be able to perform therapeutic embolization of tumours which are not accessible to any other form of treatment.

Transient ischaemic attacks

This is a clinical diagnosis. Radiological examination should start with non-invasive techniques: first, a CXR, which may show evidence of a cardiac source for emboli. A CT scan of the head will detect tumours such as meningiomas which can produce a clinical picture indistinguishable from TIAs, and ultrasound of the neck vessels may demonstrate atheromatous plaques around the bifurcation of the common carotid artery in addition to documenting the presence of any significant stenosis.

If a stenosis is present and surgery is being considered, angiography will be indicated to give a more detailed demonstration of the anatomy and to detect any other areas of atheromatous disease in the affected vessel. Arterial injection is preferable, but in some circumstances an intravenous DSA study (p. 22) will be adequate.

Suspected multiple sclerosis

MRI is now the examination of choice.

Headache

We refer here to those patients where headache is the only significant symptom, and there is no clinical evidence of intracranial pathology. We frequently receive requests for a skull X-ray in these patients, and you need to be very clear about your reasons for such a request.

If you think the headache is an indicator of intracranial disease, then the patient needs a CT scan regardless of the plain film findings. If you are happy on clinical grounds that a scan is not indicated, then neither is a skull X-ray. There is no harm in a single lateral view to reassure an anxious patient, as long as you do not allow yourself to be reassured by a normal radiograph when neurological symptoms or signs are present.

Epilepsy

CT will be indicated, particularly in adult onset epilepsy, and it also has a role in childhood epilepsy which is resistant to control

—especially when surgical treatment is contemplated. This is one area where the new scintigraphic methods for mapping cerebral blood flow may find a place. Plain skull films are almost invariably requested, but make no useful contribution. As in the case of suspected cerebral tumour, remember to obtain a CXR.

Salivary gland disease

Intermittent pain/swelling. Plain films will reveal any stone with significant calcium content, but sialography (see p. 141) will be indicated to demonstrate the anatomy of the duct system, and the presence of non-opaque calculi.

Mass. Plain films are unlikely to contribute much. Ultrasound or CT should be the initial investigation. Sialography is unlikely to add any useful information.

Sinusitis

This is usually managed without recourse to imaging. Plain films are probably requested too often, but can be useful in difficult or resistant cases. Any suggestion of complications such as mucocele or osteomyelitis will be an indication for CT or MRI scanning. This will also be the case when sinus views suggest the presence of tumour.

It is not possible to differentiate reliably between infective and allergic aetiology on radiographic grounds.

Otitis media

See p. 127.

Thyroid disease

See p. 94.

Head and neck malignancy

CT and, more recently, MRI scanning, have become the methods of choice for diagnosing and staging head and neck cancer, and also for planning therapy and monitoring response to treatment.

11

Endocrine and lymphoproliferative disorders

In the first section, thyroid disease is considered in some detail reflecting its relatively high prevalence. An outline of imaging methods is given for the other endocrine glands.

Endocrine disease

Thyroid

Diffuse goitre. Initial investigation is biochemical, (thyroid dysfunction is considered below). In the euthyroid patient imaging has little to offer. Ultrasound will demonstrate whether the goitre is genuinely diffuse or multinodular if there is any clinical doubt.

When the patient is complaining of stridor, plain films of the thoracic inlet are usually requested to document any narrowing or displacement of the trachea. If plain films or clinical examination suggest retrosternal extension, then scintigraphy will indicate if the tissue is of thyroid origin, and CT will define the anatomical relationships of the mass.

Clinically solitary nodule. There are conflicting opinions on the most suitable imaging sequence, but the aim is to ensure that we miss as few malignancies as possible, while at the same time avoiding the removal of benign lesions. Fine needle aspiration biopsy (FNAB) is beginning to assume a central role in the management of thyroid nodules, and some workers have suggested that it is the only investigation required. However, most of us feel that imaging still has an important role to play.

Ultrasound is the most sensitive technique for determining whether a nodule is truly solitary or simply one of many in a multinodular gland, but its importance in differentiating between cysts and solid masses has been over emphasized, as very few thyroid lesions are purely cystic. Isotope scanning, using ^{123}I or technetium, is nearly as good at diagnosing multinodularity, and has the additional advantage of showing if the nodule is functioning or 'cold'—malignancy is more likely in cold nodules. Even so, most solitary nodules are cold, and most cold nodules are benign, so a further weeding out process is needed before submitting patients to surgery, and this is when FNAB should be performed.

Thyroid dysfunction

Hypothyroidism. The diagnosis will usually be reached on the basis of clinical features and hormone and antibody levels, and imaging will seldom be contributory.

Thyrotoxicosis. Ultrasound has little to offer, but scintigraphy is useful in distinguishing between Graves' disease and toxicosis due to solitary toxic nodule or toxic multinodular goitre. This distinction can have implications for treatment. Some clinicians now feel that it is important to distinguish between functioning nodules which are still under pituitary control and those which are autonomous and likely to lead to toxicosis. Scintigraphy following T_3 suppression is helpful in sorting these out, although a sensitive TSH estimation will frequently be enough to distinguish between them. Discuss difficult cases with your radiologist or nuclear medicine physician.

Iodine uptake estimations are performed relatively infrequently, having been largely replaced by the battery of thyroid function tests now available. Still useful occasionally though, for example in cases of toxicosis due to thyroiditis, where the uptake will be paradoxically low.

Localization of ectopic thyroid tissue. Ultrasound or CT/MRI are the methods of choice for characterizing any soft tissue masses and defining their relation to surrounding organs. However, to prove that the lesion is functioning thyroid tissue, scintigraphy is required. This will also tell you if there is any functioning thyroid tissue in the neck.

Suspected thyroglossal cyst. Unlike ectopic thyroid tissue, thyroglossal cysts are characteristically cold on scintigraphy, but ultrasound will confirm the presence of a mass and demonstrate any cystic element.

Thyroid cancer. The role of ultrasound and scintigraphy in diagnosing thyroid malignancy has been covered above. Briefly, malignancy typically presents as an ultrasonically solid lesion with reduced isotope uptake. There are ultrasonic features which suggest malignancy, but none of the imaging appearances are sufficiently specific to determine treatment, and FNAB or surgery will be the final arbiter.

Whole body scintigraphy using radioiodine has a role in detecting metastases in patients with known thyroid malignancy. However, metastases take up considerably less activity than normal thyroid tissue, and there is no point asking for a scan unless all normal thyroid has been ablated, and thyroid replacement therapy stopped to allow TSH levels to rise. This will usually require that the patient be transferred from T_4 to T_3 for three weeks, and all replacement stopped for ten days prior to scanning. Even then, only metastases from tumours with a follicular element show appreciable uptake.

Standard bone scintigraphy is also useful in detecting skeletal metastatic disease.

Parathyroid glands

The simplest investigation of the parathyroid glands is undoubtedly high frequency ultrasound scanning. Modern ultrasound equipment produces high spatial resolution images of superficial structures and many centres report good results in detecting enlargement of the parathyroid glands. This can be augmented by ultrasound-guided aspiration of suspected parathyroid adenomata, either for cytological confirmation or parathormone assay. CT has not proved particularly effective in demonstrating parathyroid enlargement, unless gross, due to limitations of spatial resolution. Some centres claim good results with MRI and this may be particularly useful in ectopic glands. Again, spatial resolution is a limiting factor.

Parathyroid scintigraphy is used for the pre-operative localization of parathyroid adenomas in patients with good clinical evidence of hyperparathyroidism. It should not be used as part of the routine 'work up' in patients with hypercalcaemia, or in patients who are not being considered for surgery.

The patient's neck is imaged following the injection of technetium (which is taken up in the thyroid) and thallium (thyroid + parathyroid). Using computer techniques, the thyroid can be subtracted from the combined image, and any parathyroid adenoma is seen as a residual focus of activity.

Pituitary gland

Pituitary disease is usually associated with enlargement of the gland although changes may be very subtle. Plain skull radiography with dedicated views of the pituitary fossa is a useful starting point as gross erosion or enlargement of the pituitary fossa may be evident. Conversely, functioning microadenomata may cause no appreciable bone changes and yet produce significant symptoms. Whatever the findings on plain radiography it is likely that the patient will require CT to establish the diagnosis and to define extent of parasellar disease.

Thin section, high definition CT is required. This is best performed in the true coronal section. Contrast enhanced techniques are usually used to demonstrate functioning pituitary tumours. It is certain that MRI will have an important role in the future, a role already fulfilled in many specialized centres.

Adrenal glands

Hyperplasia and primary tumours of the adrenal glands cause a spectrum of endocrine disorders. Imaging is best reserved for those cases in whom the suspicion of adrenal disease is supported by biochemical or hormonal findings. It is much less rewarding to initiate imaging without this evidence. The adrenal glands are also a fairly common site of secondary deposits, particularly from primary carcinoma of the bronchus.

Although ultrasound may demonstrate adrenal enlargement, particularly of the right adrenal gland, which is easier to image, CT is the current investigation of choice. Contiguous thin sections are required to ensure that the whole gland is adequately imaged, allowing for minor changes in position that may occur with respiration. CT has the added advantage of being able to image paraaortic and retroperitoneal tissues, for example in the detection of ectopic phaeochromocytoma. MRI, if available, is also valuable.

Arteriography and venous sampling are still occasionally used although largely supplanted by CT. The results are often difficult to interpret and there is a significant risk, particularly with arteriography, of causing inadvertent infarction of the adrenal gland.

Adrenal scintigraphy requires different techniques to image the cortex and medulla of the adrenal.

Cortex. The pharmaceutical used is a cholesterol derivative labelled with ^{75}selenium. This is taken up into the steroid synthesizing pathway and can be used to identify adenomas or hyperplasia of glucocorticoid- (Cushing's syndrome) or mineralocorticoid-producing cells (Conn's syndrome). Consult your radiologist/nuclear medicine physician prior to booking, as the imaging sequence will extend over several days, and suppression of pituitary ACTH secretion with dexamethasone will need to be arranged.

Medulla. We use ^{123}I or ^{131}I-labelled MIBG (metaiodobenzylguanidine) which is treated by the gland as an amine precursor.

Its main use in adults is in the localization of phaeochromo-cytomas, and it is particularly useful for the 10 per cent of tumours which arise outside the adrenal, and which can there-fore be missed on CT and ultrasound. Scintigraphy also has a role in detecting metastases from malignant phaeochromo-cytomas. Again, imaging will be continued for up to seven days, and thyroid blocking agents will be required—consult your radiologist.

In children, the technique is used in the detection and staging of neuroblastomas.

These are expensive and time-consuming procedures and should only be performed as part of a planned imaging strategy in patients with good clinical evidence of adrenal disease—they are not screening tests.

Pancreatic endocrine tumours

See GIT section, p. 45. Pancreatic endocrine tumours are sometimes part of the MEA (multiple endocrine adenomata) syndrome. In this context, imaging of multiple endocrine glands may be necessary and a plan of investigation should be discussed with your radiologist.

Ovaries

Suspected ovarian pathology will be an indication for ultra-sound (transabdominal or transvaginal) in the first instance. For ovarian malignancy, see p. 72.

Testis

See p. 69.

Haematological/lymphoproliferative disease

This is a very broad topic covering both adult and paediatric medicine. Although text books have been written on the subject, we will only make a few basic comments. In new cases, the initial diagnosis may be suggested by radiological/imaging findings.

However, the main thrust of imaging is directed towards the determination of the extent of disease and the monitoring of response to therapy.

Hepato-splenic involvement

Ultrasound is a useful primary investigation in determining enlargement of the liver and spleen. Liver volume estimation is somewhat subjective but serial measurements can be made. Splenic size is more readily estimated, usually by serial measurements of axial length.

Focal lesions within liver and spleen, for example in lymphoma, can also be demonstrated by ultrasound, though CT is generally better as it also demonstrates the extent of lymphadenopathy and hence is frequently used as the primary investigation. Obviously, there is no point in requesting ultrasound if CT is also to be performed.

Lymphadenopathy

CT is the examination of choice for the demonstration of thoracic and abdominal lymphadenopathy. It is far superior to chest X-ray in delineating mediastinal disease and to ultrasound in demonstrating abdominal lymphadenopathy, particularly in the retroperitoneum. (These comments also apply to lymphadenopathy related to metastatic disease, particularly where there are therapeutic implications e.g. metastatic testicular tumour.)

Serial CT scans are performed frequently in the follow-up of patients with haematological disease, particularly lymphoma, where management is governed by the response to treatment. In the future, MRI will undoubtedly play a central role in the diagnosis and follow-up of patients with lymphoma, thus reducing the considerable radiation dose associated with serial CT scans.

Lymphangiography (see glossary, p. 139) is now seldom used, having been replaced by CT in the staging and follow-up of lymphoma and testicular cancer. The nuclear medicine equivalent, lymphoscintigraphy (glossary, p. 139) is a much simpler technique albeit with inferior anatomical resolution.

Haematological disease is often manifest in many systems and detailed considerations of imaging are outside the scope of this book. Frequently these diseases are treated in specialized units. If you work in such a unit there will be protocols to guide the investigation and management of these complex cases.

12

Vascular imaging

This section deals with imaging of the vascular tree—venous and arterial. The division between emergency and non-acute imaging is often not well defined and depends upon the clinical presentation.

Venous system

Lower limb thrombosis (DVT)

Emergency investigation may not be required as, unless the patient is at risk of bleeding, heparinization may be safely instituted prior to imaging, which is needed promptly but not urgently. It is not just the presence of thrombus, but also its extent which needs to be established, as many clinicians do not instigate full anti-coagulation for calf thrombosis confined below the knee.

In most hospitals in the UK the standard investigation is lower limb venography (see p. 143). The venous systems of the calf and thigh are demonstrated and an attempt is made to visualize the iliac veins. The diagnosis is confidently made if thrombus is outlined by contrast. If thrombus is extensive there may be under-filling or absent filling of the deep veins, the contrast being carried in the peripheral venous system. This is good indirect evidence of deep venous thrombosis, even if no clot is demonstrated. In this situation no contrast may be seen in the femoral or iliac veins and so information about the extent of actual thrombus is reduced.

In some centres enthusiastic radiologists use ultrasound imaging with Doppler and colour flow instead of venography. The results are comparable and often give better assessment of thrombus in the femoral and thigh vessels. You will soon know if your radiologists prefer ultrasound.

Radiologists, like anaesthetists, do a lot of venepuncture and are quite good at it. Nevertheless it can be extremely difficult to cannulate a vein in a grossly oedematous foot and multiple attempts at puncture are extremely distressing for the patient and staff. The dorsum of the foot is not a nice place for an injection. You can help by ensuring that the leg is elevated and bandaged prior to the examination. Do not send the patient to the radiology department on a chair with the leg dangling. A trolley or a straight leg support on a chair is sensible and humane.

Upper limb thrombosis

This is a less common clinical entity than lower limb thrombosis but conversely may require more prompt investigation and thrombolytic treatment. Venography is performed via a hand or forearm vein in a way analogous to lower limb venography. Some radiology departments use DSA and are able to reduce the total amount of contrast medium used.

Caval obstruction

Often a sinister clinical presentation, this needs prompt investigation. Contrast injections via upper or lower limbs can be used to confirm obstruction/compression of SVC or IVC respectively, but seldom give insight to the cause unless there is intraluminal disease, which is less common than in the limbs.

SVC obstruction. A chest X-ray is mandatory as the demonstration of gross pathology may avoid more time-consuming imaging techniques and urgent treatment may be necessary—often based upon presumptive diagnoses. CT is of great value in demonstrating not only the site of obstruction but the extent of mediastinal or thoracic disease. Dynamic CT scans using intravenous contrast via upper limbs can often demonstrate the level of obstruction with great accuracy.

IVC obstruction. To obtain adequate opacification of the cava, contrast may have to be given from both legs or even via the femoral veins. Venography can be complemented by ultrasound, particularly if the obstruction/compression is at hepatic or renal levels. Detail below this may be obscured by bowel gas, and CT will be required.

MRI using fast scan sequences can be very effective in demonstrating abnormal vascular flow (see below). When widely available, MRI is likely to play an important role in investigating caval obstruction.

For suspected caval obstruction a plan of investigation is required and you should consult your radiologist before initiating investigations.

Caval filters

The indication for this procedure is recurrent pulmonary emboli in the presence of adequate anti-coagulation or where anti-coagulation is contra-indicated. A catheter is introduced via a femoral or jugular vein approach and a filter extruded from the catheter into the inferior vena cava, below the level of the renal veins. The filters come in various forms but are basically a meshwork of fine metallic filaments that expand to grip the walls of the cava, forming a barrier to the passage of further emboli to the heart and lungs. Most modern filters are permanent, and the incidence of complicating caval obstruction is low. If both femoral or iliac veins are occluded by thrombus, a jugular approach will be necessary. Consult your radiologist.

Arterial system

Acute imaging

Acute arterial occlusion. The acutely cold, white limb is a true emergency and must be dealt with accordingly. Be sure you are clear at the outset which treatment alternatives are being considered. For example it is not in the patients' best interest to have a diagnostic study and then to be referred back to the radiologist an hour later for dissolution therapy. (The radiologist may not be too happy either.) Conversely, surgery without delay may be more appropriate than imaging in some cases.

Arteriography is the examination of choice. (See glossary.) If DSA is available in your hospital then it is possible that this will be performed by the intravenous route, but many studies are performed intra-arterially. The radiologist aims to show the site of occlusion and infer the cause. Dissolution therapy using urokinase or streptokinase may be employed and this is most effective if delivered by catheter on to or into the thrombus. The aim is to lyse the clot and re-establish patency of the vessel. If thrombus complicates an atheromatous narrowing, this must be dealt with either by angioplasty or surgery.

There is no doubt that in the future MRI will have a major impact in vascular imaging. Fast scan sequences are already available which permit imaging of the major thoracic and abdominal vessels and recently cerebral and peripheral circulations. If and when MRI is available to you, your own radiologists will make you aware of these innovations as they occur.

The aorta

1. Dissection. CT, MRI or angiography (performed by a radiologist) or transoesophageal ultrasound (usually performed by a cardiologist) give accurate information concerning the presence and extent of dissection. Recent evidence suggests that transoesophageal ultrasound is the most sensitive of these techniques. The diagnosis of dissection may be very difficult, and in cases

with high clinical suspicion of dissection several of these techniques may be necessary. The choice of examination may be dictated by your cardiothoracic surgeons, who often need to know the exact site of dissection to plan surgery. CT is performed using a dynamic protocol with intravenous contrast medium and the length of a dissection flap can be accurately mapped out from the thoracic aorta down through the abdominal aorta. Angiography requires rapid sequence techniques or the dissection flap may be missed, but has the advantage of allowing examination of the coronary arteries in dissection involving the aortic root.

2. Leaking aneurysm. CT (or MRI) is often used in preference to angiography. The presence of peri-aortic disease in leaking aortic aneurysm can be well documented and the extent of involvement of the abdominal aorta and the iliac segments demonstrated. More precise information concerning involvement of visceral and splanchnic vessels is obtained on angiography. Although extremely useful in the diagnosis and monitoring of abdominal aneurysm (see cold imaging section, below), ultrasound is of limited use in the acute phase.

3. Aortic trauma. This topic is covered in the trauma section. In summary, CT is the investigation of choice in the abdominal aorta as it is an effective, non-invasive method of demonstrating the aorta and adjacent tissues. Angiography is usually preferred to investigate trauma to the thoracic aorta.

Obviously you will need to consult with the radiologist or cardiologist concerning the acute investigation of these serious conditions.

Cold imaging

1. Arterial insufficiency. The information requested by investigation may be either anatomical or physiological or both. The standard investigation and often the only one available to you is arteriography. This demonstrates anatomical disease: stenosis, distribution of atheroma, collateral circulations etc.,

from which flow will be inferred. Although we most commonly investigate the aorto-iliac-femoral-popliteal circulations, the same general principles apply to mesenteric, carotid and upper limb circulation.

Some centres use Doppler ultrasound to obtain physiological data about blood flow. Computer analysis of blood flow spectral wave-forms can demonstrate velocity changes and turbulent flow associated with stenoses and give reproducible data concerning limb blood flow. This is therefore a useful method of following up patients with arterial disease e.g. after surgery or angioplasty, as well as giving additional information about the physiological significance of lesions demonstrated by primary investigation. Nuclear medicine procedures can also give accurate estimates of limb blood flow in these patients—consult your radiologist.

As mentioned above, MRI will undoubtedly play a major role in the future evaluation of peripheral vascular disease.

2. Aortic aneurysm—diagnosis. In this section concerned with non-acute imaging we are essentially discussing the diagnosis of aortic aneurysm and the monitoring of any changes that occur, particularly in size or extent, which may precipitate surgical intervention.

Many thoracic aortic aneurysms are diagnosed from the plain chest X-ray, but in the elderly, where considerable unfolding of the thoracic aorta may occur, definite diagnosis may be difficult from the CXR alone. Contrast enhanced CT or MRI are able to clearly demonstrate the extent and dimensions of thoracic aneurysms in cases of doubt.

The examination of choice for diagnosing and monitoring abdominal aortic aneurysms in the quiescent phase is ultrasound. Although gas often precludes optimal visualization of the abdominal aorta, it is usually possible to get enough information from ultrasound about the calibre of the aorta and relationship of any aneurysm to the renal arteries and the bifurcation.

The exact criteria for monitoring and intervention will be governed by the surgical practice in your hospital. There is an argument for early surgical intervention in aneurysms with a diameter greater than 4 cm as the natural history of the disease is for the aneurysm to increase in size and eventually rupture or leak. If you intend to treat surgically, aneurysms demonstrated on ultrasound should be further examined by angiography to delineate their extent with particular reference to the renal arteries. Intravenous DSA studies are often adequate, avoiding the necessity to catheterize the aneurysm. If the aneurysm is less than 4 cm in diameter, follow-up ultrasound is performed, usually at a time interval of approximately 6 months.

13

Trauma

Since all trauma implies some degree of urgency, this chapter will be divided into skeletal and non-skeletal injury, rather than emergency and 'cold' imaging. We are not intending to provide an exhaustive account of the radiology of trauma, rather we are attempting to outline the important general principles and highlight areas where there are particular points to be made about the role of imaging in management.

Skeletal trauma

General principles

Choice of investigation. For the majority of suspected fractures the only imaging required is plain radiography of the area in question. Those cases where things are not quite so simple will be covered in the specific injuries section (below).

Priorities. The specific fractures and dislocations covered below are considered as if they were isolated injuries. You should remember that in the severely injured patient the treatment priorities and sequence of investigations will often be dictated by coexisting soft tissue and visceral injury (see specific injuries section, below).

Importance of adequate radiographs. You will need two views of suspected fractures, preferably at right angles, if you are to avoid mistakes: even then, we have all seen occasional examples where the break was only visible on an oblique projection. The radiographer will normally perform the right views for you, and will give helpful advice if you feel that further films might be useful. In some patients the pain or immobility resulting from the injury will make it impossible to obtain the ideal projection, and compromise will be required. It is always risky to exclude a fracture if, even for the best of reasons, the films are inadequate. If in doubt, treat as a fracture until you can take advice, ortho-paedic or radiological.

When doubt persists. If clinical suspicion of a fracture is high but the radiographs are normal, treat appropriately and repeat the films in a week or so. When repeat views are inconclusive, or it is difficult to obtain satisfactory plain films, consider scinti-graphy. A normal bone scan 48 hours or more after the injury virtually excludes a fracture. But please, only do this if the result will affect management.

Comparison views. These are often requested to assess difficult areas such as the immature elbow. However, comparison views can cause more problems than they solve, since few patients are completely symmetrical, and they will often be unnecessary if you are able to obtain a radiological opinion on the initial film.

Radiographer reporting. This is not the place to discuss the role of radiographers in reporting casualty films. However, an experienced radiographer has a lot to offer the puzzled junior doctor (by way of film interpretation, we mean), and a com-promise which has been reached in many departments, including ours, is the 'red spot' system. When the radiographer examining the patient thinks an abnormality is present, a 'red spot', or some other marker, is stuck on the radiograph in question. Most junior doctors find this a help, and audit has demonstrated an improvement in diagnostic accuracy where this system is used. The important points to remember are:

1. Radiographers are just as fallible as the rest of us—films without a 'red spot' must be viewed just as carefully as those with one.

2. The radiographer may have 'seen' something that isn't there. When in doubt, discuss the film with them.

3. The 'red spot' may be there to indicate an abnormality other than a fracture—this is commonly the case with CXRs. Again, when in doubt, discuss the film with the radiographer.

Specific injuries

1. Head injury. The important clinical decision to make in head injury is whether there is any evidence of intracranial damage—patients never (well, hardly ever) die of skull fracture alone. Where there are signs or symptoms of neurological damage, the patient will need a CT scan; if this requires transfer to another hospital, it will seldom be justifiable to delay the process while plain radiographs are obtained.

Because casualty officers are understandably concerned at the possibility of sending a patient home with an undiagnosed skull fracture, routine skull radiography in virtual every patient complaining of head injury, however trivial, has unfortunately become the norm.

In an attempt to reduce reliance on the skull X-ray for medico-legal purposes, the Royal College of Radiologists, in conjunction with neurosurgeons, has drawn up guidelines for the use of radiography (Table 13.1).

2. Spine. Plain films of the suspected fracture site will be the first investigation, but in potentially unstable injuries there will often be difficulty in obtaining adequate films. The radiographer will do the best that he or she can, but when there is any doubt about the presence of a fracture, or when a fracture has been diagnosed but more information is required about its stability or associated neurological injury, CT or MRI is indicated.

Either CT or MRI or both should be available in major trauma centres, and will frequently be the initial investigation, offering considerably more information than plain films without the need to move the patient.

In isolated fractures of the transverse processes of the lower thoracic or upper lumbar vertebrae, consider the possibility of

Table 13.1   Guidelines for the use of skull radiography in
head injury (RCR 1989)

Radiography is recommended in the following circumstances:

1. Suspected penetrating skull injury or FB

2. Patients with the following signs or symptoms:
   - blood/CSF from nose or ear
   - haemotympanum or bleeding from ear
   - loss of consciousness, however brief
   - focal neurological signs or symptoms

3. Head injury plus other trauma implying a particularly strong force
   of impact.

---

associated renal trauma (see section on non-skeletal trauma
below).

3. Ribs. A CXR and possibly oblique rib views will clearly be
indicated in patients with major chest injury. The vast majority
of requests for rib views, however, are in patients who have
suffered minor trauma only, often some days previously. If they
are otherwise fit and well, the presence of the odd cracked rib
will make no difference to management and the temptation to
request radiography should be resisted.

Remember that fractures of the upper three ribs should lead to
a search for neurovascular injury.

4. Sternum. The important point about suspected sternal
fracture is that it is a difficult bone to image using plain
radiography. It is not seen at all on the frontal CXR, and the
standard views are the oblique and lateral. Even then, you may
be in doubt, and if the presence of a fracture will influence
management, CT is indicated.

As with fractures of the upper ribs, associated visceral injury
may well be more important than the sternal fracture itself.

5. Shoulder dislocations. Plain films will confirm the clinical diagnosis and, more important, exclude the presence of a fracture. Beware the uncommon posterior dislocation in which the AP film may look almost normal—the axial view (either directed up at the axilla with the film above, or vice versa) is particularly important in these cases. If it is not possible to move the arm sufficiently to obtain an axial projection, the radiographer will do their best to get a transthoracic lateral view. This should not often be necessary, as it is possible to obtain an axial view with as little as 15° of abduction.

6. Elbow trauma. Really only included to emphasize the point made in the general principles section concerning comparison views. They will seldom be required. Fractures around the elbow in children are easily missed, including some which need surgical treatment, for example avulsion of the medial epicondyle. When in doubt, immobilize the arm and bring the patient back when a radiologist is available, rather than performing lots of unnecessary views.

7. Scaphoid fractures. Remember that radiographs taken at the time of injury can be normal, so when doubt persists, re-examine in a week or ten days and repeat the X-ray if necessary. This is an area where bone scintigraphy can be useful. A normal scan at 48 hours or more post-injury excludes a fracture.

8. Internal derangement of the knee joint (IDKJ). The most you will see on the plain films, unless there is an associated fracture, is an effusion. These patients need arthroscopy and/or arthrography. This is an area where MRI will have a part to play. In centres lucky enough to have easy access to a scanner, it will replace the other techniques in at least some patients.

9. Ankle injuries. Not all ankle injuries require imaging (see requests to avoid section, below). However, major ligament tears can cause even more long-term disability than straightforward fractures. One approach is to obtain stress views. The object is to reveal any instability of the talus in the ankle mortice. This may necessitate infiltration of the suspect ligament with local anaesthetic, and will certainly require the presence of a doctor to perform the stress. This may involve you—find out what the local policy is in your hospital.

Requests to avoid

1. Isolated nasal bone. If there is no deformity, and if there is no suspicion of associated fractures in other facial bones, the presence of a crack in the nasal bone will not influence treatment.

2. Minor rib. See specific injuries section, above.

3. Lumbar spine in acute back strain. More is said about this elsewhere (Chapter 9), but remember that young fit patients do not fracture their spine by lifting a heavy weight.

4. Ankle injuries. Radiography of the ankle accounts for much of the work in our casualty X-ray departments, and a lot of it is unnecessary. There is general agreement that patients who can bear weight, and where examination shows no bony point tenderness, can safely be treated as soft tissue injuries (but see also specific injuries section, above).

5. Terminal phalanx. 'Stubbed toe, ? fracture' is a request familiar to all radiologists. Most casualty reporting piles contain several of these. Like the nose and ribs, an isolated crack in a terminal phalanx is irrelevant—the treatment is that of the soft tissue injury. The only possible exception is where the skin is broken, raising the possibility of a compound fracture. Even here, radiography is only relevant if prophylactic anti-infection measures would be instituted in such a case.

Non-skeletal trauma

Introduction

Cases of visceral trauma are often complex, with injuries to multiple organs and associated damage to the musculo–skeletal system. Investigation in such cases needs to be dictated by the clinical status of the patient and the priorities of the injuries.

Below is an alphabetical list of organs, briefly listing the diagnostic pathways in suspected trauma. Some conditions are considered elsewhere, and the page reference is given.

Aorta—abdominal

The need for intervention may preclude any investigation. For example, a patient with clinical signs of intra-abdominal bleeding, failing to stabilize on conservative measures, may require urgent laparotomy. CT, usually with contrast enhancement, is probably the most effective non-invasive method of demonstrating the aorta. If CT is not available, angiography can be employed, and with DSA the intravenous route can be used, avoiding the need to catheterize the aorta. Angiography has advantages over CT in that it better demonstrates injuries to associated major vessels, especially the renal arteries. Ultrasound (although helpful in delineating trauma to solid viscera) is unlikely to give useful information about aortic trauma.

Aorta—thoracic

A chest X-ray may reveal widening of the mediastinum and associated pleural fluid. However, rapid sequence angiography is the investigation method of choice, and the supervising radiologist will endeavour to show at least the roots of the great vessels arising from the arch as these are damaged in approximately 5 per cent of cases of aortic trauma. Radiological signs of mediastinal haematoma as demonstrated on CXR or CT may not relate to aortic or arterial damage and are frequently due to venous bleeding within the mediastinum. Angiography and CT will aim to show the site and extent of aortic damage. Trans-oesophageal ultrasound is becoming more widely available and is very valuable in suspected aortic dissection (see p. 105) but less appropriate in aortic trauma, where the patient's condition is unlikely to permit endoscopy.

Brain

Skull X-ray may indicate fractures, but the presence or absence of fractures does not necessarily correlate with underlying brain damage (see skeletal trauma section, above). CT is the investigation method of choice, demonstrating a wide spectrum of cerebral trauma, not only extra- and intracerebral collections of blood, but also cerebral contusion, oedema, and basal skull fractures.

Bladder

Cystography is the examination method of choice and is usually performed via an indwelling catheter. Transurethral catheterization may be hazardous as crush injuries of the pelvis are frequently associated with trauma to the urethra, commonly a shearing of the urethra from the bladder base. Therefore, if there has been any problem in catheterization, the urethra must be examined first (see below). Ultrasound may suggest bladder injury by the presence of fluid in the pelvis but this is non-specific and could be blood from another site. IVU may be helpful, but can appear normal in the presence of significant bladder trauma.

Diaphragm

A frequently overlooked injury in cases of severe trauma, and often diagnosed late. The chest X-ray may show disruption of the diaphragm with gut in the thorax, especially the stomach which may obstruct. Non-ionic or isotonic contrast medium needs to be instilled either orally or via a naso–gastric tube. If there is associated thoracic trauma with blood in the thorax, the exact position of the diaphragm may be extremely difficult to elucidate. Ultrasound and CT, particularly with sagittal or coronal reconstructions, may be useful.

Eye

Many orbital injuries are associated with skull or facial bone fractures. They may be difficult to diagnose from plain films, and tomography or CT are often required. Ophthalmic ultrasound may be available in your hospital. This is a highly specialized investigation method but can be extremely accurate in demonstrating conditions such as dislocation of the lens, retinal detachment or localizing intraocular foreign bodies.

Gut

Plain abdominal films may show signs of enteric perforation. Contrast examinations are not rewarding and laparotomy is likely to be necessary. Bleeding into damaged gut or from splanchnic vessels is investigated by angiography or scintigraphy.

Kidneys

The IVU is one first-line investigation method. Renal trauma may be indicated by extravasation of contrast or by failure of opacification if there has been damage to the renal pedicle. The IVU is sometimes used to show that the other kidney is functioning and apparently normal. This is a crude indicator, but is effective in emergency situations.

Ultrasound is good for demonstrating visceral trauma and, in particular, perinephric haematoma or disruption of the renal capsule. However, ultrasound may underestimate the severity of renal trauma, as bleeding can, in the early stages, be isoechoic with the surrounding renal parenchyma. There is therefore a case for both IVU and ultrasound in the investigation of acute renal trauma. Your hospital may well have a protocol. CT, with its superior contrast resolution will often be better than ultrasound in delineating the extent of parenchymal trauma and perinephric collections.

If there is clinical suspicion of damage to the renal pedicle, or absent function on the IVU, then angiography or isotope studies should be performed to see if the kidneys are perfused. Nuclear medicine studies have the advantage of documenting function although angiography is better at demonstrating the anatomy. Obviously bleeding from a ruptured renal pedicle can be catastrophic and there may be no time to instigate imaging.

Don't forget that both ultrasound and CT are also useful in looking for trauma in adjacent organs for example, liver or spleen.

Liver

Ultrasound is the most easily performed initial investigation but a better appreciation of extent of injury can usually be obtained by CT. However, if ultrasound has demonstrated significant liver damage there is little to be gained from CT in initial management.

Lungs

Chest X-ray is the initial investigation method. Pneumothorax is a common complication of thoracic cage injury. If there is a significant pneumo-mediastinum, consider the possibility of ruptured bronchus. Lung contusion shows fairly typical appearances of initial consolidation of a non-anatomical distribution which clears centrally, sometimes giving the appearance of pseudo-cavitation. CT is the second-line investigation method and gives a good overview of all thoracic structures.

Oesophagus

Chest X-ray may show widening of the mediastinum or a pneumo-mediastinum but the diagnosis of tear/rupture requires installation of non-ionic contrast medium to demonstrate the site and extent of any leak. The radiologist will be careful to avoid using barium, as leakage can result in a severe mediastinitis.

Pancreas

Often injured in rapid deceleration injury for example, seat belt trauma. Ultrasound may demonstrate oedema or even disruption of the gland, but often in severe trauma the patients' condition mitigates against a good demonstration of the pancreas in its entirety. Contrast enhanced CT (see acute pancreatitis, p. 5) will demonstrate damage to the gland and make an accurate assessment of viable pancreatic tissue. Duct disruption may only be inferred by ultrasound or CT and is confirmed by ERCP, usually at a time when the patient's condition has stabilized. Remember that the duodenum is frequently involved when the pancreas is severely traumatized.

Spleen

Ultrasound is a useful primary investigation method but more complete information can be expected from CT. Some centres report good results from using isotopes, but CT, preferably with intravenous contrast enhancement, remains the preferred investigation.

Testis

Ultrasound is the primary investigation method. Clinical management hinges around disruption of the capsule, and most cases of testicular trauma with no significant capsular disruption are managed conservatively. Colour-flow Doppler gives a good indication of perfusion to the testis, and infarction is a well recognized complication of severe trauma. If total infarction is suspected this can be confirmed by perfusion scintigraphy.

Urethra (see bladder above)

Frequently associated with fracture/dislocation of the pelvis. Following rupture the proximal and distal ends of the urethra may separate and retract. The distal urethra is assessed by ascending urethrography. If no contrast reaches the bladder and complete disruption is suspected, then a descending urethrogram via supra-pubic catheter will be necessary to demonstrate the proximal urethra and the distance between the separated portions.

Vascular

Trauma to the aorta has been discussed above but do not forget that trauma to smaller vessels can be just as catastrophic if not attended to quickly. The medical defence organizations' publications frequently remind us that arterial trauma associated with skeletal injury can be overlooked. Arteriography is required (assuming immediate surgery is not vital) and transcatheter arterial embolization is a useful treatment option for example, in cases of pelvic trauma.

Severe trauma

This chapter can only aim to give broad guidance. If this seems like a 'cop out' it is because we cannot hope to cover the complexity and wide variation in the presentations of severe trauma. Only in specialized centres where resuscitation, imaging and surgery are closely integrated can be ideal be approached. You must assess the situation quickly and instigate only those investigations that are vital to the immediate management of the patient.

Let us assume the patient's condition is stable. Plain films can usually be performed in the resuscitation area of the A and E department. Decide upon those investigations that are vital now and get them all performed quickly, accepting that they may be suboptimal and difficult to interpret. Leave those that are not vital until later—you will not want to use up valuable time and the results will be better. If you think visceral trauma has occurred, alert the radiologist as soon as possible so that he/she can organize the investigations. Often the situation is unclear. Ultrasound (and this can be performed in the A and E department) is a quick and easy way of assessing the abdomen. Clear evidence of visceral trauma may be demonstrated and the presence of blood in the abdomen indicates that significant trauma has occurred. Even if this is non-specific it may guide the surgeon to the approximate location of the source of bleeding.

Above all don't jeopardize the patient by inappropriate investigations when the attentions of a surgeon or neurosurgeon are required.

14

Paediatric imaging

When it comes to imaging, children are not just small adults, they fall prey to different diseases, and even basic investigations such as the barium meal and enema will call for different techniques to those used in adults. Paediatric radiology is a sub-specialty in its own right, and a book like this cannot pretend to cover the field—in particular, we have not attempted to deal in detail with the special problems of neonates.

We stay with the format used in most of the other chapters, picking out for inclusion clinical conditions which could present to the junior hospital doctor in A and E or outpatients.

Remember that radiation protection is especially important in children—their tissues are more sensitive to the effects of irradiation, and they have the whole of their lives ahead of them in which to manifest any ill effects.

Remember too that young children may not be able to co-operate to the extent required even for fairly simple procedures, and sedation is sometimes needed. Sedation is very much a two-edged sword though, and can cause more problems than it solves, so always discuss cases with your radiologist where there is any doubt about the need for it.

Emergency imaging

Acute upper airway obstruction

A child presenting with signs of severe upper airway obstruction is unlikely to require any imaging procedure until the airway has been safeguarded, which may of course involve endoscopy under anaesthetic or even tracheotomy.

Children with less critical symptoms should have a lateral soft tissue view of the neck and a CXR. These films can be very difficult to interpret in sick unco-operative children, and a radiological opinion should be sought as soon as possible.

The four diagnoses most likely to underlie this clinical presentation are viral infection (croup), acute epiglottitis, retropharyngeal abscess, and inhaled foreign body (covered separately below). Our aim is not to teach interpretation of films, especially in such a difficult area as this, but a few specific points are worth making

1. Croup is usually a viral infection. Any airway narrowing visibly in the films tends to be at and below vocal cord level. The radiographs may be normal.

2. Acute epiglottitis is a serious condition, and you will know all about the dangers of injudicious clinical examination of the pharynx. The lateral soft tissue view is the important one, and will show oedema of the epiglottis and surrounding region. Remember that any necessary radiography should be performed as quickly and with as little fuss as possible. As mentioned above, the suspicion of acute epiglottitis will often lead to examination by an anaesthetist without recourse to imaging.

3. Retropharyngeal abscess produces widening of the retropharyngeal soft tissues, sometimes gas is seen within the swelling. A difficult diagnosis for the inexperienced, as similar soft tissue widening can be produced by forward flexion of the neck and expiration (especially if the child is crying).

Inhaled foreign body

Many inhaled foreign bodies are non-opaque, peanuts being the classic example, and the radiographs may be normal. It is important to obtain chest films in inspiration and expiration as the only evidence of bronchial obstruction may be air-trapping on the affected side. Where the child is too young to co-operate, the radiologist will need to screen the chest to assess volume changes during respiration. When suspicion persists in spite of normal imaging, or when the diagnosis is confirmed by the radiographs, the patient will need bronchoscopy, and further radiological investigation will not be indicated. When the neck and chest films are normal, and depending on the nature of the foreign body, you may need an abdominal film in case it was swallowed rather than inhaled. Always do the chest/neck films before the abdomen, otherwise you can miss a foreign body which is on the way down!

Acute asthma/status asthmaticus

The CXR may be normal—its value lies in the exclusion of complicating factors such as pneumonia or pneumothorax (see also cold imaging section, below). Prompt treatment will take precedence over radiography, which may not be necessary in cases which respond rapidly.

Acute abdomen

The list of possible diagnoses in a child with an acute abdomen will depend not only on symptoms and signs, but also on the age of the patient. In most cases plain films of the abdomen will be requested, but are of limited value. They may reveal abnormal calcification, for example, renal calculi, or signs of intestinal obstruction. Remember that it is not unknown for chest conditions (e.g. basal pneumonia) to present as abdominal pain.

Ultrasound and/or contrast studies will often be needed, and in some cases the radiological procedure itself can be therapeutic; for example, barium or air enema in intussusception.

Do not be reassured by an apparently normal plain film—involve your radiologist sooner rather than later.

Suspected acute appendicitis

The diagnosis is usually made on clinical grounds. The abdominal X-ray is unlikely to be helpful, showing only non-specific changes. A recent development is the use of ultrasound to diagnose acute appendicitis. The right iliac fossa is scanned using gradually increasing compression to displace mobile bowel loops from under the ultrasound transducer. The diagnosis is made by demonstrating a blind-ending tubular structure, with or without an appendicolith. Good results are obtained in expert hands, and if you have a paediatric radiologist, this technique may well be employed in your hospital.

Vomiting/feeding problems in the young child

In the young infant you will want to exclude pyloric stenosis. Many radiologists are now happy to make the diagnosis on the basis of the ultrasound findings, without resorting to contrast studies. You will soon discover which examination your radiologist favours. When test feeds and ultrasound are negative or inconclusive, barium will be indicated to look for gastro-oesophageal reflux/hiatus hernia, in addition to confirming normality of gastric outflow (see also 'feeding problems' in cold imaging section, below).

Finally, remember that vomiting/abdominal pain in these young children can be due to disease outside the gastrointestinal tract, for example, UTI and raised intracranial pressure.

Suspected bone/joint infection

Septic arthritis and osteomyelitis are considered together as they may coexist, and the initial symptoms and signs may be poorly localized. The important point to make is that although plain films will be the first investigation, they will be normal, or show only very subtle abnormalities if the illness is caught early enough. The gross radiological changes of osteomyelitis should be a thing of the past given prompt diagnosis and antibiotic treatment.

Scintigraphy is the investigation method of choice when bone sepsis is suspected. It is much more sensitive than radiography. Confirmation that a scan abnormality is in fact due to infection may require aspiration or biopsy.

The hip joint is one of the more common sites for sepsis, and ultrasound should be requested at the same time as plain films, as this can show the presence of an effusion when radiographs are normal. This does not prove infection of course, but again, fluid can be aspirated for definitive diagnosis.

Bone and joint infection can lead to severe disability if not diagnosed early, and investigation should be initiated on the first suspicion of sepsis.

Non-accidental injury (NAI)

This may be a clinical diagnosis, radiography simply being used to confirm the clinical impression and document the extent of skeletal injuries. Often though, it will be a suspicious finding on a radiograph which first alerts the clinician.

In either case, the investigation of choice will be carefully performed plain film radiography. The temptation to make do in small children with a 'babygram' (one or two films covering the whole body) should be resisted. Some of the radiological findings in NAI are subtle, and require good high definition films of the suspect areas if they are not to be missed. As there are few if any features which are specific to NAI, the diagnosis rests on patterns of injury, and the demonstration of fractures of differing ages.

Bone scintigraphy has a role in detecting injuries in areas which are difficult to examine on plain films, for example the ribs, but it would not normally be used as the primary imaging technique.

Sadly, some of these children will have symptoms or signs of cerebral or visceral injury, and ultrasound and CT will have a role to play.

'Cold' imaging

Heart murmurs/congenital heart disease

Although we cannot deal in detail with the investigation of childhood heart problems here, it is worth pointing out that this is one of the areas where non-invasive imaging has made an enormous impact. While neonates and infants with complex anomalies may still require cardiac catheterization, many of these young patients can be fully investigated using plain radiography, echocardiography, and nuclear medicine studies.

In older children with murmurs, echocardiography will pick up septal defects and valvular lesions, while scintigraphic techniques will give functional information such as shunt size and ejection fraction. It looks as if MRI will have an important role here, and may well be able to combine multiplanar anatomical information and quantitative blood flow data.

Ear nose and throat disease

Such common childhood problems as otitis media, glue ear, and tonsillitis will usually be managed without recourse to radiological investigation. In the case of chronic middle ear infection/mastoiditis plain films will usually be performed. The lateral view of the nasopharynx is particularly useful in children, showing any encroachment on the airway by adjacent soft tissue swelling, notably of the adenoids.

When complications such as cholesteatoma are diagnosed or suspected clinically, and plain films are inconclusive, then high resolution CT or MRI scanning is the investigation method of choice.

Any suggestion of intracranial extension of infection, or dural sinus thrombosis, will be an indication for urgent CT or MRI scanning.

Chest infection

Most chest infections in children are treated on clinical grounds. When radiography is performed, it is important to remember that a normal CXR does not exclude an acute infection. If the CXR does reveal radiological signs of infection, treatment can still be monitored clinically. A single follow-up film is more than adequate in an otherwise fit child who makes a full recovery:

certainly multiple radiographs during and after treatment are not indicated.

Asthma

The role of the CXR in asthma is to diagnose complications such as infection or pneumothorax. Regular radiography in asthmatic children as a 'routine follow-up' is unacceptable (as are such requests in most other conditions). The CXR in asthma will frequently be normal, but may show evidence of hyperinflation and/or bronchial wall thickening.

Feeding problems

This is a rather vague presenting symptom, but it is included here as it is frequently seen on imaging requests, usually where gastro-oesophageal reflux and/or aspiration is suspected. Although pH measurement is probably still the gold standard, contrast studies (using dilute barium or non-ionic water-soluble media) are the first-line imaging investigation method, and will demonstrate whether or not the child has a hiatus hernia. Remember that reflux is an intermittent phenomenon. If you feel sure an infant is refluxing, but the barium meal is normal, scintigraphy can be useful. Imaging can be continued for an hour or more in different positions, without increasing the radiation dose, and reflux can be reliably detected.

Scintigraphy is unfortunately rather less sensitive in picking up aspiration into the bronchial tree, but a positive result is useful in children with recurrent chest infections, or coughing/cyanosis during feeds.

Failure to thrive

This will often be associated with feeding difficulties (see previous section). Apart from this, it is not possible to set down a screening protocol for such a nebulous clinical entity. Do guard against the blunderbuss approach, requesting a whole host of imaging investigations in the hope that one will hit the mark (see Chapter 1). Liaise with the radiologist and try to work to some sort of logical strategy, guided by any localizing symptoms and signs that may be present.

Urinary tract infection

There are two reasons for diagnosing and treating childhood urinary tract infection (UTI). The first is to relieve the acute symptoms and rid the urine of bacteria: the only investigation required for this is an MSU. The second reason is to detect any remediable underlying cause for the infection, and prevent permanent damage to the kidneys—the condition we used to call chronic pyelonephritis, but which is now known, perhaps more accurately, as reflux nephropathy. This is where imaging comes in.

The visible sign of renal damage is focal loss of cortex, or scarring. The causative agent is almost certainly the reflux of infected urine into the kidney, hence the name reflux nephropathy. Whether reflux without infection can cause scarring remains a source of debate, but it is now accepted that the damage is done early on in life, certainly before the age of five in most cases.

When to investigate. It is generally accepted that all childen with a proven UTI should undergo radiological investigation: the only argument concerns the best imaging sequence.

Which investigation? A plain abdominal film and an ultrasound scan are adequate as first-line examinations in children over the age of two. The aim is to detect stones and/or obstruction. Further investigation will be required in infants, and in older children whose screening results are abnormal or who suffer recurrent infection.

The precise sequence of tests differs between centres, and you will need to follow your hospital's protocol. For this reason, we

will not go into too much detail, although a few general points
are worth making:

1. Where the presence of vesico-ureteric reflux will influence
   management, micturating cystography (MCU), either radiographic or scintigraphic, is indicated (p. 140).

2. Scarring may be apparent on ultrasound, but is best assessed
   with a DMSA scan, which also allows an estimate of split
   renal function. Note that acute infection can result in
   transient abnormalities of DMSA uptake, and so scanning
   should be postponed for at least six weeks following diagnosis
   and treatment.

3. Where any of the other tests have raised the possibility of
   obstruction, isotope renography is the investigation of
   choice.

Overall, the tendency is to minimize the use of the more
unpleasant and invasive techniques. In particular, the IVU now
plays a very small role in the investigation of these young
children, having been largely replaced by ultrasound and nuclear
medicine techniques.

Non-specific abdominal pain

Children presenting in this way are frequently over-investigated.
If the child is otherwise well, and clinical examination normal, it
is unlikely that any imaging procedure will advance the diagnosis.
In particular, IVUs, barium studies, and even plain abdominal
films performed on the off-chance that they will reveal pathology
are unacceptable in the absence of relevant clinical features.

When symptoms are particularly severe or persistent, and
certainly if the child becomes unwell, ultrasound is the examination of first choice. It is non-invasive, no ionizing radiation is
involved, and it allows a comprehensive survey of all the intra-
abdominal viscera. In older girls, it will exclude gynaecological
pathology. The need for other examinations will depend on the
ultrasound result and the developing clinical picture. The scan is
often curative!

Gastrointestinal bleeding

This is not a common presenting problem in children, and when it does occur, investigation will be along similar lines to that in adults (Chapter 6).

One of the more frequent causes of bleeding in children is a Meckel's diverticulum, and here an isotope scan can be helpful. We rely on the fact that Meckel's diverticula bleed because they contain ectopic gastric mucosa, which takes up pertechnetate. Consequently, any focus of uptake which cannot be accounted for by stomach or excreted urinary activity is likely to represent a diverticulum, in the appropriate clinical context.

There should be few false positives with this technique, but false negatives do occur, and so a negative scan in a patient with persistent symptoms does not exclude the diagnosis.

When you feel that a Meckel's is still a possibility in spite of negative or equivocal scintigraphy, a small bowel barium study will usually be the next line of investigation, although the diverticulum is easily missed among the ileal loops, even by an experienced radiologist. Occasionally selective arteriography will be required, but only in very difficult cases and after considerable discussion.

Musculoskeletal symptoms and signs

This chapter cannot cover all the musculoskeletal problems of childhood, any more than Chapter 9 can comprehensively deal with adult orthopaedics and rheumatology. We only discuss those conditions which are specific to childhood and where there are useful points to be made about the role of imaging. For example, juvenile chronic arthritis is not mentioned specifically, as the imaging sequence will be similar to that in adult RA.

Any musculoskeletal ache or pain in childhood which is persistent, particularly when it is severe enough to interfere with normal activity (other than school!) should be taken seriously, and will usually require imaging of some kind. Unlike adults, there is quite often a treatable cause for the symptoms, and delay can result in long-term disability, or worse in the case of primary bone tumours.

Back pain. Any non-trivial back pain in childhood will be an indication for imaging—initially plain radiography. The desire to reduce irradiation needs to be balanced against the risk of missing serious pathology, including infection or tumour.

When plain films are normal but symptoms remain worrying, scintigraphy is indicated. A normal bone scan will virtually exclude significant pathology.

If the plain film findings are non-specific, or if radiographs are normal but the scan shows a hot spot in the spine, then CT or MRI scanning is the procedure of choice, and will often allow you to identify the nature of the pathology. It also delineates the location and extent of the lesion more accurately than any other technique, and if necessary will allow guided percutaneous biopsy.

Spina bifida occulta. You will often come across this term in X-ray reports. It refers to an ossification defect in the neural arch of one of the lower vertebrae, usually around L5, and it is a very common finding. In the absence of neurological deficit or associated skin lesions (e.g. dimples or tufts of hair) it is an incidental finding of no significance.

Suspected congenital dislocation of the hip (CDH). The suspicion of CDH will usually be raised at routine clinical examination of the neonate. Ultrasound is the investigation method of choice, as it demonstrates the cartilaginous femoral head and other components of the joint. If skilled ultrasound is not readily available, then an AP film of the pelvis will usually be all that is required. A film taken with the hips abducted to 45° in internal rotation (the Von Rosen view) allows an assessment of alignment, but this is seldom necessary, and should not be requested routinely.

In older children, radiography will be used to check that the hips are developing normally following treatment. However, follow-up films should be kept to an absolute minimum, as it is possible to accumulate an unacceptable radiation dose over the years.

Hip pain. A common problem, and remember that hip disease can present as pain in the knee in childhood. The initial investigation method will be plain radiography. In irritable hip, and in the early stages of other hip disorders, radiography will be normal.

It is important, particularly if slipped femoral epiphysis is a possibility, to obtain a lateral view of the hips in addition to the AP projection. This can also be helpful in the early stages of Perthe's disease, where the changes may be subtle. Be sparing with follow-up films in order to minimize radiation dose to the gonads.

When the clinical diagnosis is irritable hip, ultrasound is the most sensitive method for demonstrating an effusion in the joint. Aspiration may be required to exclude infection, as the imaging findings can be identical (see emergency imaging section, above). In any patient with normal films, but significant symptoms, an isotope bone scan is indicated.

Knee pain. Plain films will be the initial investigation, and in the majority of cases will be normal. As always, significant persistent symptoms will be an indication for scintigraphy. A couple of points concerning specific conditions:

1. Osgood-Schlatter's disease. Essentially a clinical diagnosis, and the only role for radiography is to exclude other, more serious, pathology. Fragmentation of the tibial tubercle apophysis can be a normal finding of no significance.

2. Chondromalacia patellae. A common cause of pain, especially in young girls. You should expect plain films to be normal.

15

Glossary of investigations

This section is intended to act as a quick reference source, explaining the essential features of examinations with which you may be unfamiliar. Indications for the investigations are not given here, but will be found in the appropriate sections of the book. Imaging methods (ultrasound, CT etc.) are covered in Chapter 3.

Arteriogram

The introduction of contrast medium into the arterial tree. Performed via a catheter inserted percutaneously, the most frequently used puncture site being the common femoral artery. From there an appropriate shaped catheter can be manoeuvred into almost any artery, including the carotids and coronaries.

Usually performed under local anaesthetic with or without sedation. Used to require (at least) overnight admission; with the smaller calibre catheters now available, more are being performed as day cases.

Arthrogram

Water soluble contrast medium is injected into the joint in question and this is often followed by the insufflation of air or CO_2 to give double contrast. Can be performed on any accessible joint, but has been most frequently used in the knee. Usually no more than mildly uncomfortable, an exception being the TMJ, where anaesthesia or sedation is required. Has been at least partly replaced by MRI where it is available.

Barium studies

See small bowel (below) and Chapter 4.

Bile reflux scan

HIDA (see below) is injected intravenously and the gamma camera positioned over the upper abdomen to detect any biliary reflux into stomach or oesophagus.

Bleeding scan

Nuclear medicine procedure to demonstrate the bleeding site in patients with unexplained GIT blood loss. Uses intravenous injection of either colloid or the patient's own labelled red cells. Less invasive than arteriography (above), and at least as sensitive in the detection of bleeding. It gives less precise anatomical information however, and will not identify the nature of the bleeding lesion.

Bone scan

A diphosphate compound labelled with technetium is injected intravenously, and imaging performed about three hours later. In some cases, additional images will be acquired during and immediately after injection to assess blood flow to the bone. A very sensitive indicator of bone pathology, but non-specific, and radiography of any hot spots may be required.

Bronchogram

The instillation of contrast medium into the bronchial tree, either by way of a cannula over the back of the tongue, or by direct crico-thyroid puncture. Now virtually obsolete, having been replaced by CT for the assessment of bronchiectasis in patients being considered for surgical treatment.

Cardiac gated scan

The patient's red cells are labelled with technetium and the gamma camera, linked to an ECG recorder, follows the passage of activity through the heart for about ten minutes per view. The change in volume of the left ventricle during the cardiac cycle can then be deduced from the changing count rate. Ejection fraction can be calculated and wall motion quantified. May be impractical in patients with a grossly irregular rhythm (e.g. fast AF).

Cholangiogram

Contrast examination of the biliary tree. There are several varieties:

1. Endoscopic retrograde cholangiopancreatography (ERCP) is performed under radiological screening control. The operator passes the endoscope into the duodenum, cannulates the papilla of Vater and injects water-soluble contrast to fill the biliary and/or pancreatic tree.

Can be used therapeutically, either alone or in conjunction with a percutaneous approach (below) to remove duct calculi and place stents across malignant strictures.

2. Intravenous. This examination became obsolete due to a number of developments, notably in ultrasound and ERCP. It also carried a higher risk of morbidity (and mortality) than other investigations using intravenous contrast media.

3. Operative. The contrast is introduced via a catheter in the cystic duct during cholecystectomy, under screening control using a mobile image intensifier.

4. Percutaneous transhepatic (PTC). A fine needle is introduced into the liver under local anaesthetic. When a bile duct is entered, contrast is injected to opacify the biliary system and images taken to demonstrate the anatomy and any obstructing lesion that might be present.

5. T-tube. Contrast is injected down the T-tube left in the common duct following surgical exploration. Usually performed about ten days post-op.

Cholecystogram, oral

The patient attends for a control film of the gallbladder area. Oral contrast medium is then given, usually in two doses, one the night before, and one on the morning of the examination. Films are taken of the gallbladder before and after stimulation with an oral fat preparation. Very few indications for this now that ultrasound has become the first line gallbladder investigation.

Dacrocystography

Demonstration of the lacrimal apparatus following the injection of contrast medium into the punctum.

DMSA scan

Renal scintigraphy using dimercaptosuccinic acid. This pharmaceutical sticks to viable renal tubule cells and provides a map of the functioning renal tissue. Imaging usually performed three hours after the injection of activity.

DTPA scan

See renography (below).

Echocardiography

Ultrasonic examination of the heart, usually including Doppler analysis. Can diagnose and quantify for example, wall motion abnormalities, valve lesions, and shunts.

Galactography

The injection of contrast medium into a nipple duct orifice prior
to mammography, usually to demonstrate duct papillomas in
patients with a blood-stained discharge.

Gallium scan

Gallium is a radioactive element which localizes in inflammatory
tissue and some tumours, particularly lymphoma. Scanning is
performed from 24–72 hours post-injection. Patients may be
given laxatives to clear excreted activity from the colon.

Gated cardiac scan

See cardiac scan (gated) above.

HIDA scan

HIDA is an acronym for a group of technetium-labelled imino-
diacetic acid derivatives used in hepato-biliary scanning. Injected
intravenously, they are rapidly excreted into the bile and thence
to the gut, filling the normal gallbladder en route.

Hysterosalpingogram

The injection of contrast medium through the cervix to demonstrate the uterus and (especially) the fallopian tubes.

Leukocyte scan

A scintigraphic technique in which the WBCs from a sample of
the patient's blood are separated, labelled, (with technetium or
indium) and reinjected to localize areas of sepsis.

Lung scan

Scintigraphic assessment of lung perfusion using technetium-labelled protein microspheres or macroaggregates, and ventilation using any one of a number of radioactive gases or aerosols. Non-invasive and safe, although right to left shunts and pulmonary arterial hypertension are relative contra-indications.

Lymphangiogram

The opacification of the regional lymphatics and nodes using an oily contrast medium. Most often used in the lower limbs with the intention of opacifying the abdominal nodes. Requires a cut-down under local anaesthetic on to a lymphatic vessel which has been rendered visible by the prior subcutaneous injection of coloured dye. A skilled and time-consuming procedure, now largely replaced by CT scanning in the staging and follow-up of lymphoma and testicular cancer, which accounted for the majority of referrals.

Lymphoscintigraphy

The nuclear medicine equivalent of lymphangiography. Much less technically demanding—the labelled colloid which is used is simply injected subcutaneously and is taken up by the lymphatics. Does not give the same anatomical resolution as the radiographic technique, but is more versatile—for example, it can be injected into the posterior rectus sheath to demonstrate the internal mammary nodes in breast cancer.

Meckel's scan

Nuclear medicine technique used to pick up ectopic gastric mucosa in symptomatic (bleeding) Meckel's diverticula. Pertechnetate injected intravenously and images acquired over 40 minutes or so. Many centres pre-treat the patients with oral cimetidine to reduce gastric secretion of activity.

Micturating cystourethrography (MCU)

The bladder is filled with water-soluble contrast medium via a catheter. The catheter is removed and screening performed during micturition to detect reflux. Images recorded on film, cine or video. Can be uncomfortable and embarrassing for the patient. See also urethrography (below).

MUGA scan

(Multiple gated acquisition)—see cardiac scan (above).

Myelogram

The introduction of water-soluble contrast medium into the subarachnoid space to demonstrate the spinal cord and nerve roots. Usually injected at lumbar puncture, although direct cervical puncture can be used when the cervical cord is the area of interest. From the patient's point of view, the only discomfort is that associated with a standard lumbar puncture. See also radiculogram (below).

Nephrostogram

Contrast is injected via a nephrostomy catheter (see p. 147) to delineate the collecting system and ureter.

Pyelogram

Direct opacification of the renal collecting system; there are three types:

1. Intravenous. See p. 33.
2. Antegrade. The renal pelvis is punctured under ultrasound guidance (as for nephrostomy, p. 147) and contrast medium injected. Films are taken to demonstrate the collecting system and ureter. See also Whittaker test (below).

3. Retrograde. Contrast injected from below through a ureteric catheter introduced at cystoscopy. May be performed in theatre or X-ray department.

Radiculogram

As for myelography (above), the examination being limited to the lumbar region. So-called because it is the lumbar nerve roots which are being imaged, rather than the spinal cord, which terminates at L1–2.

Renogram

Nuclear medicine scan using hippuran, DTPA or, most recently, MAG3. Pharmaceutical injected intravenously with the gamma camera situated posteriorly over the renal area. Activity is rapidly excreted by normal kidneys, and dynamic images (e.g. 120 fifteen second images over 30 minutes) acquired on computer. Computer-generated regions of interest are then drawn over the kidneys, and time–activity curves produced. Intravenous frusemide is often given to ensure good flow rates and assess washout in suspected obstruction.

Sialogram

Demonstration of the parotid or submandibular duct system. The duct orifice is identified and dilated, contrast is injected via a cannula. Mildly uncomfortable for the patient.

Sinogram

Injection of contrast medium into a sinus opening on the body surface. Demonstrates the size and position of any abscess cavity, communication with bowel etc.

Small bowel studies

The opacification of the small bowel with barium, or occasionally other contrast media. Can be introduced by drinking (small bowel meal) or via a tube passed into the duodenum beyond the duodeno–jejunal flexure (small bowel enema). Both techniques have their enthusiasts, and both will give satisfactory results. Can be a prolonged examination and involves a significant dose of radiation. It is not possible to perform a good quality small bowel study during the same session as a double contrast barium meal, and so 'barium meal and follow-through' is no longer a valid request.

Thallium scan

Thallium is a radioactive potassium analogue, and is taken up by myocardium in addition to many other tissues. The patient is stressed, either on a treadmill or pharmacologically using intravenous dipyridamole, and the thallium is then injected. Images are acquired in three projections immediately after stress, and again at rest, approximately three hours later. Non-perfused regions of myocardium show as cold spots, and reversible ischaemia can often be differentiated from infarction by comparing stress and rest images.

Thyroid scan

Scintigraphic imaging of the thyroid following the injection of either technetium or an iodine isotope. You must let the radiologist know if the patient is on thyroid replacement treatment; this will need to be discontinued, as will some types of anti-thyroid medication. Also, remember that administration of iodine-containing contrast media (usually in the course of a CT scan or IVU) can suppress thyroid uptake, and so investigations need to be scheduled with this in mind.

Urethrogram

Contrast examination of the urethra; there are two routes.

1. Ascending. Contrast is introduced into the penile urethra using either a small balloon catheter lodged in the navicular fossa, or a mediaeval device known as the Knutsson clamp. Delineates the length of the urethra, and contrast will eventually reach the bladder. Shows the anterior and bulbar urethra nicely, and also the lower end of any stricture. Doesn't provide very good distension of the posterior urethra, and can be difficult to get past a tight stricture. Therefore usually combined with:

2. Descending. As for MCU (above). Films taken to show the urethra during micturition. Delineates the proximal end of strictures and gives better distension of the posterior urethra.

Urography

See IVU, p. 33.

Venogram

Usually lower limb, looking for evidence of a DVT. A tourniquet is placed at the ankle, and contrast injected into a vein on the dorsum of the foot. Films taken to demonstrate the deep veins of the leg, thigh and pelvis. Also used in the upper limb when axillary vein or SVC thrombosis is suspected.

V/Q (V/P) scan

See lung scan (above).

Whittaker test

As for antegrade pyelogram (above). Fluid is infused into the renal collecting system at a constant rate, and pressure is monitored. An abnormal rise in pressure is an indication of obstruction.

16

Glossary of interventional procedures

This section gives you some information about the more common interventional procedures performed by radiologists. You may not find all these procedures available in your hospital. A number of specialized interventional procedures, only performed at a few centres, have been omitted.

The introductory remarks concerning the role of the clinician are only a general guide, and if you are in any doubt about the preparation of patients or their aftercare, we recommend that you find out from your radiologist what is required.

Clotting screen

Frequently the radiologist will want to see an up-to-date clotting screen, including platelet count, prior to the procedure. Blood will need to be cross-matched for some of the more invasive procedures.

Consent and pre-medication

This should be the responsibility of the radiologist performing the procedure. If possible, the radiologist will try to see the patient on the ward to explain what is involved, to answer questions and generally allay anxiety. He/she will be in a far better position than you to answer the patient's questions and obtain informed consent. Due to the pressures of time upon us all, this consent may be obtained in the radiology department just prior to the procedure. You should not instigate pre-medication on your own initiative if consent has not been obtained. The radiologist cannot obtain informed consent from a sedated patient. Under special circumstances, usually a frequently-performed procedure for a specialized unit, good quality informed consent may be obtained by the referring clinicians, but this should only be done with the full knowledge and acquiescence of the radiologist.

Aftercare

Following the procedure the radiologist may need considerable help and co-operation from you and your ward staff in the aftercare of the patient. For example, surveillance of the limb following angioplasty, or ensuring the security of external drainage catheters. Be sure that you know what is required and if necessary get further information from the radiologist. We would rather discuss the case with you than have to deal with the complications of mis-managed aftercare.

Angioplasty

This is the dilatation of vascular strictures, usually arterial. The radiologist negotiates a balloon catheter through the stenosis or occlusion and, by inflating the balloon within the narrowing, dilates the stricture. It has a high success rate with low morbidity and has replaced surgery as the number one option in many patients, particularly in the coronary, renal, iliac, and lower limb circulations. The risks mainly relate to damage of the vessel at the time of balloon inflation.

Biopsy

Biopsy guided by imaging has had a major impact on patient investigation in recent years. Commonly using ultrasound or CT for guidance, the radiologist can accurately direct a needle (either cutting for histological specimens or fine needle for aspiration cytology) into abnormal tissue. The main associated risks are those of bleeding or damage to adjacent structures, but using imaging guidance, major structures can be avoided and these risks significantly reduced. Your radiologist will usually ask you to obtain an up-to-date clotting screen on the patient before performing biopsy.

Drainage

Abscess

Using imaging guidance (ultrasound or CT), fluid collections and abscesses can be drained percutaneously. This can be performed either by inserting a sheath, performing the aspiration and withdrawing the sheath, or leaving an indwelling drainage catheter *in situ*. Access, avoiding surrounding major structures, is the important factor, and in difficult cases CT is usually better than ultrasound in determining the route for drainage.

Biliary

Many obstructed biliary systems are now relieved by the retrograde insertion of a stent at ERCP (see stenting below). Sometimes this is not possible and external percutaneous biliary drainage is performed by the radiologist via the lateral or anterior approach, using fluoroscopy or ultrasound for guidance. The radiologist opacifies the biliary tree by inserting a fine needle and injecting contrast medium. Using a combination of sheathed needles, dilators and guide wires the biliary tree is catheterized. If a biliary obstruction can be negotiated, a prosthesis (stent) is inserted percutaneously through the stricture and into the duodenum to permit drainage of bile—internal drainage. If this is not possible, a catheter is left within the dilated duct system and bile is drained through it—external drainage.

Renal—nephrostomy

Obstructed kidneys can be drained by the percutaneous insertion of catheters into the dilated upper renal tract and urine drained externally. This is usually performed under ultrasound guidance although in some centres fluoroscopy is also used. Remember that nephrostomy may not be appropriate if the renal obstruction is due to stone disease, and you are planning to treat the stones by lithotripsy. Many lithotriptor machines involve the use of a heated water bath. The nephrostomy is effectively an open wound and cannot be placed in the water bath, which is a good bacterial culture medium! In this situation, retrograde insertion of ureteric stents via cystoscopy is the preferred option. External drainage by nephrostomy can be converted to internal drainage by antegrade insertion of ureteric stents (see below).

Embolization

This is the occlusion of vessels by the introduction of thrombogenic foreign material via a catheter.

Arterio-venous malformations (AVM)

Only performed in specialized centres but consult your radiologist anyway as he will probably know the expert to whom you can refer your patient.

Bleeding

Arterial embolization is a useful alternative to surgery in some cases of arterial bleeding, for example an inoperable renal tumour causing persistent haematuria or internal iliac artery bleeding in severe pelvic trauma. Embolization of solid viscera is often associated with significant post-procedural morbidity: commonly fever, pain, and leukocytosis. Bleeding from the portal venous system can be treated by transhepatic portal vein catheterization and embolization of varices. This is a very specialized procedure not available in all radiology departments.

Venous

There is sometimes a need for venous embolization for example, large varicoceles. This is often a very effective alternative to surgery and can be repeated if collateral circulations develop.

Stenting

A stent is a semi-rigid tube, introduced across strictures to restore or maintain patency.

Biliary

This has been referred to above in biliary drainage. Stents are introduced either percutaneously or at ERCP. A recent innovation is the use of expandable metal stents within the biliary tree as an alternative to smaller calibre plastic stents. The wider calibre obtained is particularly useful in bile duct malignancy. Such stents can also be introduced retrogradely by the endoscopist.

Renal tract

Antegrade stenting can be performed as a sequel to nephrostomy (see above). A guide wire is negotiated down the ureter and into the bladder and a soft, double J or double pigtail catheter inserted to effect internal drainage. This can be useful in cases where retrograde stent insertion is not possible for example, when a bladder tumour overgrows the ureteric orifices. Unhappily in cases of diffuse pelvic malignancy the patency of such stents is often short lived.

Vascular

As described above in biliary stenting, a recent innovation is the use of expandable metal stents. These intravascular metal stents can be used in various situations within the arterial and venous tree and there is some evidence that the restenosis rate is significantly reduced compared to straightforward angioplasty. The two disadvantages are the possible interference with subsequent surgery, and the extremely high cost of the stents.

Stone removal

Gallstones

Most gallstones left in the bile duct at routine cholecystectomy are removed endoscopically with sphincterotomy and stone extraction. If this is not possible and a T-tube is *in situ*, calculi can be removed percutaneously via the T-tube track. The track is usually left to mature for 4–6 weeks and then the stone is removed by a basket inserted along this track under fluoroscopic guidance. It is a great advantage to the radiologist if the T-tube is brought out laterally as this will enable him or her to manipulate whilst avoiding the primary X-ray beam.

A recent vogue has been the percutaneous removal of gallstones from the gallbladder, usually a combined procedure involving radiologist and surgeon. The gallbladder is punctured percutaneously and a sheath inserted through which an endoscope can be passed to remove the gallstones. In many centres this technique has been superseded by the advent of laparoscopic cholecystectomy.

Renal

Only performed in a few specialized centres and largely replaced by lithotripsy, this technique involves the percutaneous puncture of the renal collecting system, the passage of an operating sheath and the removal under direct vision of the calculi.

Thrombolysis

Recent thrombus can be dissolved by the insertion of a catheter
into the appropriate vessel and the instillation of streptokinase
or urokinase. (See vascular section.)

Vena cava filters

See vascular imaging section, p. 104.

17

Glossary of radiological terms

**Terms used more frequently by radiologists
than clinicians**

Artefact

An apparent abnormality on a film which is actually unrelated
to anything within the patient (e.g. marks due to processing).
Also used in a more specific sense, for example movement
artefact (blurring!).

Amorphous

Lacking any recognizable structure or pattern. For example,
amorphous calcification, as opposed to punctate or 'popcorn'
calcification.

Attenuation

Absorption of the X-ray beam as it passes through tissues.
Varies according to the physical properties of the tissues. Mainly
CT term.

Companion shadow

A line seen paralleling the border of a rib or clavicle, and due to
normal adjacent soft tissue structures.

Composite shadow

An apparently abnormal opacity which, when analysed, can be accounted for by the superimposition of normal structures.

Consolidation

The mention of consolidation in a CXR report is often taken to mean infection. However, the term simply indicates that air-containing lung has been replaced by fluid. This may be pus, oedema, blood, or inhaled stomach contents. The same optical density may be produced by solid tumours.

Decubitus

See under 'projection' below.

Density

Describes the relative attenuation of a structure, for example 'a low density lesion'. Used for ionizing radiation hence X-ray or CT, but not ultrasound or MRI.

Dose

Amount of X-ray radiation absorbed by the patient.

Echogenicity

(Reflectivity.) The degree to which an organ or tissue produces echoes on ultrasound scanning. In the appropriate clinical context, the degree of echogenicity of a lesion can enable the ultrasonographer to differentiate between various pathological processes. The same concept is conveyed by the term 'echo amplitude'.

Echo-poor

Reduced echogenicity.

Geographic

Description of a type of bone destruction with clearly defined margins—indicates a mildly/moderately aggressive process.

Honeycomb

A confusing term, now largely abandoned. Appearances of criss-crossing linear fibrosis on chest X-ray. Does not correlate with pathology and is unhelpful.

KUB

A plain abdominal film taken to cover the <u>k</u>idneys, <u>u</u>reters, and <u>b</u>ladder, usually looking for renal tract calcification or calculi.

Lytic

Used to describe an area of bone destruction, for example by tumour or infection.

Miliary

A CXR appearance consisting of multiple, small, well-defined pulmonary opacities. Examples are miliary TB, sarcoid, and metastases.

Moth-eaten

Multiple 'holes' in an area of bone destruction—indicates moderately/severely aggressive process.

Nephrogram

The phase in the IVU when the kidney parenchyma is demonstrated immediately after the injection of intravenous contrast medium. Due to capillary and early tubular opacification.

Osteopenia

Radiographically demonstrable bone demineralization—does not indicate a specific cause.

Penetration

(Over/under) Refers to the degree of exposure (blackening) of the film: underpenetrated = underexposed (too white), overpenetrated = overexposed (too black). Overpenetration, if not too severe can be overcome by viewing the film against a bright light.

Permeative

A diffuse, poorly defined destructive pattern (of bone)—indicative of an aggressive condition—malignancy or infection.

Projection

The relationship between X-ray tube, object, (patient) and film. The aim is to choose a projection which puts the region of interest as close to the film as possible, to minimize magnification and blurring.

AP/PA (antero-posterior/postero-anterior). In an AP projection, the film is behind the patient, and the X-ray tube in front. For a PA the positions of tube and film are reversed. In other words, the AP/PA refers to the direction travelled by the X-ray beam relative to the patient. The CXR is routinely performed PA, ensuring that the heart is closest to the film, thus reducing magnification and movement artefact (see above).

Left and right lateral. Hopefully the 'lateral' is self-explanatory. The left and right refer to the side which is placed nearest the film; so, when a CXR shows an opacity at the right base, you will want a right lateral and vice versa.

Decubitus. The patient is examined lying on their side (right side for right decubitus and vice versa). A horizontal X-ray beam is used, and this is a useful alternative to erect films in demonstrating fluid levels/free gas when patients are too ill to stand. Also performed as a routine in the double contrast barium enema.

Lordotic. Used mainly for lung apices on chest X-ray, occasionally to demonstrate fissural pathology. AP projection with patient leaning back at 20°.

Punctate

Usually of calcification: small (<1 mm), clearly defined.

Reflectivity

See echogenicity, above.

Reticular

CXR pattern reduced by overlapping linear fibrosis. A preferred term to 'honeycomb'.

Septal lines

(Kerley's lines.) Small peripheral linear opacities on the chest X-ray indicative of fluid in the peripheral lung interstitium. Most commonly seen in LVF but may also be present in other conditions such as resolving pneumonia or lymphangitis carcinomatosa.

Sclerotic

Increased bone density (i.e. whiter than usual on the X-ray)—
the opposite of lytic (above). May be generalized, as in some
dysplasias, or focal, for example in metastases from prostatic
cancer. It is a non-specific response of bone to a number of
different physiological and pathological stimuli, often represent-
ing an attempt at repair.

Signal

Now an MRI term. Indicates the information received by the
detectors at the completion of an echo sequence. It is this
information that is computer processed to produce the images.
Hence 'high signal' or 'signal void'.

Trans-sonic

Describes tissue which transmits the ultrasound beam well,
giving rise to few, if any, echoes. Typically seen in fluid-filled
structures, for example, simple cysts or a full bladder.

Unfolding

The opening-out of the aortic arch seen in hypertension and
arteriosclerosis. Can be considered a normal finding in the
elderly.

References

Beir, V. (1990). *Health effects of exposure to low levels of ionizing radiation*. National Academy Press, Washington, D.C.

Grainger, R.G. (1984). The clinical and financial implications of the low-osmolar radiological contrast media (letter). *Clinical Radiology*, **35**, 251–252.

Grainger, R.G., and Dawson, P. (1990). Low osmolar contrast media: an appraisal. *Clinical Radiology*, **42**, 1–5.

Jacobson, P.D., and Rosenquist, C.J. (1988). The introduction of low osmolar contrast agents in radiology: medical, economic, legal, and public policy issues. *Journal of the American Medical Association*, **260**, 1586–1592.

Katayama, H., Kozuka, T., Takashima, .T., Matsuura, K., and Yamaguchi, K. (1988). Adverse reactions to contrast media: high osmolality versus low osmolality media. Scientific exhibit. Radiological Society of North America, Chicago.

RCR (Royal College of Radiologists) (1989). *Making the best use of a department of radiology—guidelines for doctors.*

RCR and NRPB Joint Report (1990). *Patient dose reduction in diagnostic radiology.* Documents of the NRPB, **1** (3).

Index